# THE
# RENEWED
# PRACTITIONER

# THE
# RENEWED
# PRACTITIONER

*How Spiritual Care Transforms Nutrition,*

*Dietetics & Lifestyle Medicine*

*Mary Gannon Kaufmann*

---

## CHAPTER 4

---

---

## CHAPTER 5

---

---

## CHAPTER 6

---

PREFACE

*Helpful Thoughts in Getting Started*

I was moved to begin this book after having conversations with a few other dietitians. I asked one whether she integrated spirituality into her practice and what barriers or difficulties she experienced if she tried to address her clients' spiritual needs. This dietitian responded readily and shared that addressing religious needs was essential to her practice. She said, "Many people come to me because I'm a faith-based dietitian. They know that I'll bring in Scripture and pray with them." When I asked about her clients who were not Christian, and she said, "I don't offer religious/spiritual care to them," I was moved to clarify how spiritual care could impact nutrition counseling and lifestyle medicine for all patients, even those from diverse backgrounds. When it comes to lifestyle medicine and nutrition, is not it essential to address many aspects of practical living and human needs as dietitians, nutritionists, and healthcare professionals?

I asked another dietitian if she considered other aspects of spiritual care outside of reading Scripture and praying with patients. Her response startled and even amused me. She wondered if I was just trying to stir controversy. My answer was yes and no. I think healthcare, including dietetics and lifestyle medicine, is being invited to grow to meet the needs of people today, from various backgrounds, who live complex lives. Many people struggle with personal or spiritual distress, to find meaning and purpose, and how to deal with unavoidable stress and negative outcomes. Providers are being asked to develop new skills to be able to offer compassionate care that addresses the needs of the whole person. Lifestyle medicine providers, including dietitians, offer much more than nutrition and lifestyle information. In the words of Dr. Daniel Salmasy, medical doctor, philosopher, and Franciscan Friar, "The patient deserves more than an automaton dispensing technology" or evidence from the literature.[1]

I realized, however, that dietitians, nutritionists, and other non-chaplain members of the healthcare team may not know what I'm suggesting: the importance of developing well-rounded intelligence like spiritual intelligence or how to recognize and address the non-tangible, existential needs in their patients, and themselves even, needs that really impact physical and mental health. We also may have some confusion about our goals as practitioners, about well-being, and health.

As an aid to this endeavor, this author has developed an interactive training program, The Renewed Practitioner Training, to assist Registered Dietitians and lifestyle medicine providers in implementing the concepts described in this book: spiritual care within their primary practices. This supportive outside training seeks to enhance the growth stimulated from this book. Another alternative to taking outside training is to read through this book with a small group of peers and work through the activities in Part Two so either way you can each review your interactions with patients, and receive constructive and supportive feedback from a facilitator and engaged peers. For information on the virtual yet live training and small groups, please contact the author and Healthy Rise Nutrition and renewedpractitioner.com.

## Defining some terms and describing the learning process

To begin, we want to define a few terms, like spiritual intelligence and the transformative learning process so you can effectively use this reference. So far, we have referred to spirituality, spiritual care, and spiritual intelligence. You may not know the difference between these terms or why describing each can impact our understanding and spiritual care (SC) of patients as we practice lifestyle medicine. Spirituality relates to having spiritual intelligence, like a noun relates to a verb. In this work, we will define spirituality as a human universal need and describe the personal and physiological impact that results if it is thwarted or stunted. We will explain how to cultivate a spiritual way of being. To be spiritually intelligent is the action and ability to "bring one's spirituality and the transcendental relationship with the sacred into daily problem solving."[2]

Spiritual intelligence was a term forged in the late 1990s as the discussion of multiple intelligences began. Intelligence is an "independent yet intertwined mental skill set that works in different dimensions of human existence."[3] SI is intelligence directed at existential matters. Researchers have deduced that SI is the personal knack for using your spiritual lens to understand deeper elements about the world, your work, and the needs of others, including what motivates them, along with the ability to expand your awareness of what makes life meaningful, your own purpose, and the capacity to have an increased spiritual consciousness.[4]

In this work, we use growing in spirituality and spiritual sensitivity as a way for a person to grow in spiritual intelligence. We use spirituality and spiritual intelligence interchangeably. By its very nature, spirituality is both a reality and an action.

Spirituality grows, as we will discuss, and it impacts how we do things, how we see the world, and how we engage with the ups and downs of life. Growing spiritually equips us to possess wisdom in caring for others, to see their needs, struggles, and potential, and to find deeper reasons for being, a greater meaning and purpose.

In subsequent chapters of Part One, you'll examine transcendence, spirituality in more detail, spiritual distress, and grief, and see the evidence of their impact on inflammation, the health of most body systems, body image, and readiness to change, to name some of the important dimensions. You will also learn why it is important for all healthcare professionals to be alert to assess and develop strategies to meet the spiritual needs of their patients as well as their own. Could this gap in understanding be the reason that, despite receiving excellent medical care, your patients may not be making the progress you have hoped for and that you, at times, may struggle with morale in your own profession?

Over the years, from the research, we see that knowing about spiritual care or just having spiritual intelligence as a practitioner is not enough to be able to offer effective spiritual care. Providers need personal formation. We describe this as transformative learning, head and heart learning, which creatively follows a model from clinical pastoral education and the CPE process that trains healthcare chaplains. Here, clinical process learning is formatted and adapted uniquely to support non-chaplain healthcare professionals, particularly lifestyle medicine providers, including dietitians and nutritionists, to grow in their capacity to incorporate spiritual care (SC) within their primary disciplines. This care is inclusive, empathetic, and sensitive to patients from different faith traditions or no faith tradition at all.

We see initially that positive spirituality is an untapped health asset, while carried grief and spiritual distress may negatively impact the best medical care. Spirituality, more and more, is being examined objectively through evidence-based research, but in many ways, it retains an irreducible mystery along with grief, well-being, and even health. Rational thought helps us understand these experiences, but part of what you will hear here is the invitation to react, reflect, and linger with what is presented. As a practitioner, you can stay centered on the evidence while you are guided from within to practice the art and craft of caring uniquely for your patients.

## How transformative learning works & how to use this reference

Transformative learning, which we will describe in Part Two of this work, is multi-dimensional and seeks movement and change, as well as to build and ground what you already know with new evidence that you can apply to your work today. It impacts your thoughts, your heart/emotions, your capacity to engage with clients on sensitive issues, and, hopefully, your perspectives on living, but it's more. It's grounded in your own life and reflections as you learn and read new evidence while considering your life and work. It is more than gaining an intellectual understanding of a new discipline—spirituality inside healthcare medicine. This dynamic process is a proven means that allows you to grow in personal insight and examine under your own hood, looking objectively and critically at how you engage with patients—their needs, hopes, and wounds—while staying cognizant of your own inner landscape. Your clients can heal more deeply while you renew your own vigor for caring for them, avoiding burnout or recharging if you've experienced depletion. Untended spiritual needs can be the loose thread in patients' lives and their health-seeking behaviors, as well as what hampers and unravels your own professional and personal well-being due to compassion fatigue or burnout. The goals are to "weave meaningful activities and situations into a daily life routine,"[5] so you can better impact the clients you serve and find deeper meaning and purpose yourself as you practice dietetics, nutritional care, or work in another healthcare profession.

To start, ask yourself this question, 'How have I noticed my own practice develop and grow? What challenges or barriers have I encountered when I work as a professional? Do I need to learn something new to be more effective, or am I burnt out and needing to recharge? Build upon your own foundation. Spirituality is a very powerful energy for living and very personal, too, impacting how you live and how you offer care to others.

Getting back to our initial reflections, yes, hopefully, this work challenges you and is somewhat provocative. With new paradigms, often there is a pull back to the familiar that can hamper growth. According to Russo-Netzer, a common temptation when something new is suggested is "to consider the status quo as a reference point to potential change and favor the current state of affairs, since the potential costs of change appear to carry more weight than the potential benefits."[6] The hope is to avoid this tendency and to awaken your thoughts and feelings as well as a new understanding of spirituality—that hidden sense in human life that motivates each person to something greater, in their being, their spirit, and their deepest meaning and purpose for living.

Right from the start, you want to be anticipating growth in yourself and your facility for working with patients on the human level. The aptitudes taught assist you in developing skills in self-reflection and self-awareness, in interpersonal lingering, in practicing real-person listening as opposed to diagnostic listening, and in companioning your patients (and yourself) in life-enhancing ways. These skills will assist you in opening up the listening session to capture the power of the patient's narrative in life reminiscence that will also empower their acquisition of healthy behaviors. Likewise, you will examine what seems contradictory, but nonetheless real: how to be supportive while being able to confront patients in ways that build trust in the caring relationship so they can flourish.

Additionally, you will learn how to manage the intense emotions that clients express. Some providers become overwhelmed by their patients' profound feelings, leading to burnout, while others act more as companions, guiding individuals to appreciate their own emotional experiences. Generally, dietitians and healthcare professionals often take on caretaking roles, making them susceptible to compassion fatigue. This training will reveal that you can provide support without becoming entangled in the pain of others.

Practicing the craft of patient care holistically brings a certain healthy humility and vulnerability to professional caregivers, which facilitates healing for patients and practitioners alike. What we are after is that "special kind of knowledge" described by Ibarrando et. al, "that allows nurses [healthcare professionals] to act in a more reflective manner and with tact and skill, in certain situations and relationships that arise in their daily practice."[7] What we describe through this work is care that respects the integral wholeness of human persons, for both patients and practitioners.

Amid the process, you will want to become aware of your own foibles so you can better emotionally support those you care for. What's more, you will come to understand that offering spiritual care to patients is more than using spiritual or religious language when talking with them, more than simply praying or engaging with a sacred text, and more than discussing their spiritual or religious beliefs.

However, once patients bring up these topics, you can engage with them in these ways. Spiritual care involves listening to the patient's narratives and often to their deepest needs in such a way that you help them tap into their raison d'être, their motivations, needs, and barriers to cultivating their health and well-being in a life well lived.

# INTRODUCTION

*The Untapped Power of*

*Spiritual Care in Nutrition*

*& Lifestyle Medicine*

Maybe you've picked this book up wondering what spirituality has to do with nutrition and lifestyle care. Some people who may be spiritual themselves feel that for a healthcare professional to address spirituality in care is unethical and outside the scope of practice unless the provider is a healthcare chaplain. They may feel unprepared. Others who try to impact their nutrition counseling with biblical principles for religious clients stop short of integrating spirituality into their practice if the person is not religious, while some speak of religious principles and irritate clients. How do we bridge this gap, or should we?

There are many references out there that, for the last 25 years or more, have been encouraging health professionals and non-healthcare chaplains to learn about spirituality and screen for spiritual distress and spiritual needs. These recommendations have been presented primarily to nurses, pharmacists, physical therapists, physicians and a few other healthcare disciplines, encouraging them to include spirituality in their patient assessments. For example, The American Medical Association passed resolution 304 (A-24) for Addressing Patient Spirituality in Medicine and stated the Association "recognizes the importance of individual patient spirituality and its impact on health, and encourages patient access to spiritual care, and promotes medical education curricula on spiritual health." Unfortunately, registered dietitians, certified nutritionists and lifestyle medicine professionals, including integrative and functional medicine providers, have been omitted or missed in these discussions.

This oversight is important to rectify, as dietitians are the healthcare professionals who spend the most time with clients. For example, according to Cohen,[8] studies show that physicians spend 17–24 minutes with a patient. Nurses see 4.5 patients per hour or spend 13 minutes per patient, while registered dietitians, according to the CMS Manual,[9] spend 45–90 minutes per patient session.

A registered dietitian and nutritionist's goal is optimal wellness to "enhance health as positive vitality."[10] As a discipline, dietitians base their care and priorities on science and evidence, while building a partnership with clients to assess their lifestyle and personal and body systems' needs. Dietitians build on what the client is doing and don't impose a value system (author's thoughts). According to Noland, the hope is to "balance the mind, body, and spirit" by using "natural, effective, less invasive interventions when possible" to allow the body's physiology and metabolism to re-equilibrate. Dietitians promote healing and prevention of disease by focusing on rebalancing nutrition and lifestyle factors, and they spend longer periods with patients to accomplish this. The emphasis is on wellness rather than simply reducing symptoms of illness, so spiritual care is a natural extension.

Most other healthcare providers lack training in these non-invasive methods of nutrition and lifestyle medicine, which, according to Kris-Etherton, have shown equal, if not superior, benefits in treating chronic and metabolic diseases as pharmacological interventions, with less risk and side effects.[11]

Dietitians apply science to nutritional care and utilize certain counseling skills, such as motivational interviewing, cognitive behavioral therapy, or acceptance and commitment therapy, to empower and engage clients in optimizing their health. Dietitians, through this lens, can develop as well-rounded practitioners by attending to the whole person, with intention, by offering spiritual care inside their discipline.

Spiritual care is an untapped noninvasive aspect of whole-person care that dietitians have not been fully aware of and has tremendous potential. In addressing spiritual needs, the RD can build deeper trust with clients and maximize their motivation and physiological health by assisting them in tapping into what matters most to them. They also can more fully understand the obstacles that their patients encounter. From observing informal discussions between dietitians in mentoring or Facebook groups, I have often seen dietitians claim that a patient's failure to implement nutritional changes was due to "low readiness to change" when, in reality, the person may have lost sight of what gives them meaning and purpose, or not found helpful ways to recharge and motivate their human spirit. As we will see shortly, positive spirituality is a very powerful health asset for all people, although everyone defines spirituality uniquely. On the other hand, spiritual distress and prolonged grieving hamper optimal health for humans, increasing stress-related illness and disordered eating behaviors or compensatory behaviors. Rather than just supporting the down and out, as spiritual care has previously been described in the healthcare literature, dietitians play a unique role in promoting whole-life wellness or spiritual vitality compared to other disciplines. Dietitians contribute a unique aspect of spiritual care in promoting spiritual wellness, with additional training and support.

Without being aware of one's own spiritual needs and experiences, healthcare professionals lack the sensitivity to pick up on subtle yet impactful clues about deeper spiritual issues that affect health. What's more, if a provider or dietitian carries unresolved or unconscious emotional baggage from their own life experiences, they may be unprepared or unavailable to welcome others into this deeper emotional space within lifestyle medicine. When the provider is uncomfortable, they divert the interaction to where they feel at ease: providing information. This powerful aspect of health and body-based wellness, spirituality, can best be supported by clinical process education, which will be discussed in the second half of this work. Without this action-reflection-action model of training, practitioners will know about spirituality but cannot truly navigate or address it with clients.

As we have described, many practitioners struggle to have a clear picture of the wholistic health that whole-person care can provide. We are so used to following the evidence of the science that we have missed forming a total picture of health. In the next chapters will explore our history and where we are headed in forming this wholistic focus in lifestyle medicine. Are we after health, wellness, well-being or forming a flourishing life? According to Pinto Teixeira, providers who are spiritually mature or possess greater spiritual intelligence are more likely to be resilient, to grow from challenges and not burn out, to engage in more principled thinking, exhibit better citizenship behavior, and demonstrate more favorable social interactions, including improved communication skills. What's more, according to research, spiritually sensitive practitioners have also been shown to have greater empathy, a capacity to forgive, higher job satisfaction, and a sense of personal ownership of their jobs while being less likely to be stressed out, depressed, or overly anxious.[12] With all the positive benefits, both professionally and personally, for all aspects of living, how could we have missed developing spiritual care training for health professionals, especially registered dietitians and lifestyle medicine professionals?

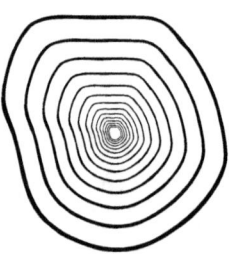

# PART
# 1

# CHAPTER 1

*Is Spiritual Care in*

*Dietetics & Lifestyle Medicine*

*Something New?*

At the beginning of the 20th century, the connection between health and spirituality was part of common thought in the medical arts until it was diverted by germ theory and the growth of the sciences.[13] This connection played a strong role in the origins of nutrition and dietetics as a means of health. If we look to earlier times, a focus on diet began with Hippocrates (460 BC) and Plato (460–348 BC), who coined the term "diet" from "the Latin *diaeta*, meaning mode of life," a word that was used in a broader sense than it is today.[14] In Greece, about the 8th century BC, physicians and philosophers described that a proper diet was a precondition for corporal and intellectual well-being."[15]

The American Dietetic Association started in 1917 with the growth in chemistry and focused on the physical needs of the body: vitamin and mineral deficiencies, for example, such as iron deficiency anemia, and later, in 1943, with the endorsement of the U.S. military, on macronutrient needs. Now, however, as penned by Professors Hwalla and Koleilat in 2004, nutritionists and dietitians are being driven by a growing public interest in nutrition – "the contribution of diet to chronic problems and the demands of an ageing society" as well as "new sources of competition from web-based information services." The field is broadening once again to consider life, a new mode in all the complexities today, including spirituality in the medical arts.

Rightly so, the field of Dietetics and Nutrition is developing, growing, and evolving. More dietitians are expanding their skills to examine personalized nutrition, root causes of health, and their roles in healthy lifestyle medicine beyond just food and culinary arts, like the faith-based dietitians mentioned in the preface, and many others are expanding their skills in the therapeutic use of self.[16]

Many are attempting to integrate into their assessments more aspects of human life and culture, clients' daily self-management habits as well as the nutritional aspects, biomedical markers and medications. According to Nagy et al, dietitians trained over the last 30 years notice the move from nutrition education to relationship building, collaboration and shared decision-making. Many, however, "do not feel adequately trained to manage the emotional aspects of the therapeutic interaction."[17]

At the foundation, and back to our origins, according to the Academy of Nutrition and Dietetics in the USA, "RDs contribute the critical thinking, code of ethics and evidence-based practice that is unique to nutrition and dietetics science and practice."[18] Swan et al. further described "nutritional and dietetics practitioners as thoughtful professionals who acquire, analyze and interpret the important and relevant data contributing to the potential nutrition-related problem or problems." Dietetics is based on evidence that is interpreted for individual people in nutrition counseling and communities in public health.

In a recent statement, however, and seemingly indicative of a more holistic emphasis on living, in the Standards of Professional Performance for Registered Dietitian Nutritionists in Eating Disorders, the Academy of Nutrition and Dietetics encourages dietitians to grow in responding to the affective needs of their patients by developing their therapeutic skills. Practitioners are "admonished to form a conscious awareness of medical, psychological, and behavioral strategies… to develop a dynamic and holistic view of ED treatment" by the RDN.[19] They are asked to "undertake ongoing self-evaluation of their skills and knowledge base, and to seek ongoing postgraduate training, supervision, and mentorship to achieve ever-growing expert practice competence for their advancement to a higher practice level."[20]

Moreover, the Academy of Nutrition & Dietetics and many training programs for dietitians and lifestyle medicine professionals encourage providers to form effective communication skills and cultivate their interpersonal qualities of warmth, care, and personal attentiveness to patients.[21] Most practitioners admit that patients respond to their warmth and speak about deeply personal concerns during sessions.

Along with therapeutic skills (like motivational interviewing, the application of cognitive behavioral principles, and more), practitioners are to augment the Nutrition Care Process. Swan describes that dietitians need to have a dynamic relationship with clients *to interact with them.* When dietitians interact with them, however, have they been considering all relevant data and parameters that are impacting the nutritional status and health of their patients? Ask yourself: do you move beyond building rapport to therapeutically linger, to support, motivate, and, at times, challenge your clients to break through the barriers to personal wellness and quality of life, including spirituality?

Are practitioners now guiding and supporting clients while they apply the science to be healthy and lead fuller lives? Can this "advancement to a higher practice level" mean more than offering spiritual care when people are down and out, to recognize the needs of the human spirit when experiencing trauma, ill health, or sadness, as some researchers exploring spiritual care within healthcare have suggested? Some also question and express doubt that all persons have spiritual needs and that, according to McSherry et al., "It should not be assumed that patients will require help from health care professionals with their spiritual needs."[22] These are questions that we hope to support you in addressing in your own life and with the patients that you serve. Could the goal of including spiritual support within the healthcare relationship be something more: to accompany the patient in forming a fulfilling, flourishing life, even in distress, difficulties, and suffering.

## Is the goal health, wellness, well-being, or ultimately, a flourishing life?

Although the terms health and wellness, or well-being, are often used interchangeably, they are best described as distinct concepts. There is a benefit to parsing out their differences, especially in trying to understand whole person-centered care and the process of behavior change. Both health and wellness are multi-dimensional terms, with well-being understood as "How people feel, how they function on a personal and social level, and how they evaluate their lives as a whole."[23] Health focuses on the more objective qualities and characteristics of a person in their body; "i.e., their biomarkers and how well their body and brain are functioning."[24]

Flourishing, on the other hand, expands health and well-being to impact the community at large. According to the Health Equity & Policy Lab at the University of Pennsylvania, "A flourishing person has the ability to help their body thrive, have their emotional needs met, possess the trust and cooperation to function in social settings, and use reason for individual and collective ends."[25] Human flourishing becomes the ultimate goal because it denotes both personal and systemic wellness and quality of life: the growth, development, and holistic well-being of both individuals and populations.[26] It seems that, often, dietitians, until now, have placed a stronger emphasis on aspects of health rather than considering pertinent influences on wellness and well-being, with the ultimate goal of supporting a flourishing life.

These concepts can be applied to spirituality and religion as well to ascertain a person's subjective experience of their spirituality, spiritual practices, religion, and religious practices that impact health. According to Kopacz et al., religion and spirituality can involve both private or personal practices (meditation, prayer, individual contact with nature, or listening to religious media) that cultivate sensitivity and personal growth, as well as public expressions of these life priorities (joining with a community in public religious practices).[27] Idler (1994) describes this religious well-being as "The outcome of religious practice, through which one attains a meaningful degree of social cohesiveness (social group involvement and support obtained from a religious group/congregation) and cognitive coherence (i.e., a religious interpretation of life's events), both helpful for buffering stress in times of crisis."[28] In fact, Kopacz found evidence for this stress-buffering effect, showing that "veterans with a self-reported history of suicide ideation had significantly lower public and private religiosity scores compared to those who did not report a history of suicide ideation."[29] Could it be that until now, when practitioners stay solely in the sciences, they have missed key aspects of well-being: spiritual practices and religious interpretation of events that have negatively impacted how their patients pursued health behaviors?

With this in mind, patients' subjective feelings toward their life and health, as well as the impact and adjustment to illness, are important aspects of care to investigate with clients if the focus is on health, wellness, and living a flourishing life. In fact, according to Hancock et al. (2012), patients desire that "dietitians know them individually, to provide personal acceptance of their feelings and needs and offer them emotional support."[30] Perhaps a patient's failure to follow through with recommendations, including implementing healthy eating and lifestyle changes even when motivational interviewing and cognitive behavioral principles are applied, is due to an imbalance—an unspoken need in an unaddressed aspect of their life: their religious or spiritual well-being. It may not be that they have a low readiness to change or a need for more information. Practitioners, however, often feel more secure and comfortable focusing on facts and information rather than feelings. When practitioners fail to hear patients on a deeper level, central motivating needs often go unaddressed and become barriers to follow-through.

There is religious and spiritual wellness, as well as well-being in physical health, which the Academy of Nutrition and Dietetics recognized in the Revised 2019 Standards of Practice and Standards of Professional Performance for Registered Dietitians

Nutritionists in Nutrition in Integrative and Functional Medicine. Registered Dietitians are to "seek a balance between mind, body, and spirit" and identify health as "positive vitality."[31] Dietitians are healthcare providers; when spirituality is integrated into care and assessment, who can promote spiritual wellness rather than just alleviate spiritual distress. This focus on vital wellness makes the dietitian's role in providing spiritual care within their discipline unique compared to any other healthcare discipline.

## A model for holistic health

Where do we look to decipher these imbalances that may be impacting our clients' wellness and health? We start by looking to organizations that promote world health for our communities and within our healthcare organizations. The World Health Organization and resolution WHA 37.13 state in the Health for All initiative that "health is a state of complete physical, mental, social, and spiritual well-being and not merely the absence of disease or infirmity."[32] This comprehensive sense of well-being came from the realization that something was missing without the spiritual aspects of the human person. Likewise, Samuel Hynd, the health minister of Swaziland and a member of the WHO who initially raised the question about spirituality and health for the Health for All Initiative, stated: "There is a dimension to a man or a woman that goes beyond and above their physical, mental, and social well-being. There is something within a person, what one could call attitude, motivation, driving force, or whatever name you call it, but which I prefer to call spirit."[33] Spirituality is this often-overlooked aspect of humanity, the essence of true health that is often overlooked, and its importance dismissed.

Investigators later characterized this driving force as "an ennobling principle" within human persons, which if overshadowed or diminished, "institutes a state of malaise that comes from seeing the person in a purely materialistic, physical perspective."[34] They describe "the spiritual aspect of life as complementary to health, care for the body and the mind, as the body, mind, and spirit are inseparable in humans and must be taken into consideration in healthcare." This sense of "something more to life" seems to surface when a person encounters something they appreciate but something also that they cannot control.

In like fashion, the Joint Commission, whose mission is to improve healthcare for the public by evaluating and credentialing healthcare organizations in the USA, requires "all members of the healthcare team to assess patients' spirituality: to ascertain and meet spiritual needs."[35] Also, another group credentialing palliative care agencies in the USA, the National Consensus Project for Quality Palliative Care, requires all healthcare providers "to develop and document a plan based on the assessment of religious, spiritual, and existential concerns using a structured instrument and integrating this information into the care plan."[36] In the same report, palliative care providers—meaning all members of the healthcare team—are asked to also address "spiritual and existential concerns that include assessing for all types of pain, psychological concerns, and grief."

These recommendations from the World Health Organization, Joint Commission, and the National Consensus Project for Quality Palliative Care sprang from the study of health psychology and lived experience. Since the 1970s, this biopsychosocial model of health psychology has been evolving and now suggests that there are limitations to promoting health when the focus is placed primarily on the physiological, psychological, or social parameters alone.[37] Important factors that motivate individuals to take care of themselves have been oversimplified. This shortsightedness obstructs the acquisition of healthy behaviors and, consequently, lasting wellness and well-being. "Spirituality, then, is meant to enhance, foster, or augment the biopsychosocial domains so that humans can have a deeper response or fuller function for health in the body, in our moods, and in relationships. It also exerts an independent effect on health by expanding a person's awareness of power outside oneself and of a deeper meaning and purpose in working through suffering and difficulties."[38]

Many within the health provider community, more in Europe than the USA, have coined and used another term to describe this integration of the body, mind, social relationships, and spirituality and its impact on health: salutogenesis. The salutogenic model of health posits that "life experiences help shape one's sense of coherence—an orientation towards life as more or less comprehensible, manageable, and meaningful."[39] The thinking is that balancing and synergizing the physical, emotional, social, as well as spiritual dimensions into a working wholeness of living brings health or wellness. Spirituality, then, becomes the grounding force, the base where humans are able to grapple and refocus in the midst of unknowns and experiences they cannot control.

Maslow, who famously formulated Maslow's Hierarchy of Needs also described that the human being requires a framework (a coherence) or "values, a philosophy of life, a religion or religion surrogate to live by and understand by, in about the sense that he needs sunlight, calcium or love."[40] When healthcare professionals practice spiritual care in the midst of their discipline, they are listening for this sense of coherence: what primary values motivate the person's pursuit of wellness and what type of support would ground them to follow through with living life. They are also listening for any ways the pursuit of this coherence and their primary values have been thwarted or burdened by loss. The thwarting relates to spiritual distress, while the burdening by loss is grief. Each can impact their freedom to pursue health-seeking behaviors and their body's physiology. Additionally, when a provider suggests a mind-body practice to rebalance the person's life, they want to keep in mind what they have discerned about these issues in the person's life, rather than suggesting a novel mind-body practice that may seem foreign to the person.

Health promotion becomes wellness and involves more than just taking medication to alleviate symptoms, correcting nutritional deficiencies with nutrients, or slapping on a novel mind-body practice. It is a dynamic process where practitioners offer individual recommendations for unique people after ascertaining their personal needs, values, and culture. To be most effective, nutrition and lifestyle recommendations need to touch on the whole: the body, the emotions, their thoughts and participation with a social group, and consequently, their vocation and their human spirit, which resonates towards something greater than themselves alone.

Notice your own responses to this discussion. Does this surprise you? Does this resonate within you as a practitioner or are you stirred and experiencing some resistance to these statements? Would you rephrase any of the words to make better sense to you?

## The importance of recognizing transcendence

To get in touch with this force inside of you—transcendence—imagine standing at the base of a mountain in Telluride, Colorado, in the Rockies, or in Lucerne,

Switzerland, in the Swiss Alps. How are you drawn to, in the words of Augustine (354), this "Beauty ever ancient and ever new?"[41] And what is your relationship in that moment to the Universe? In this light of salutogenesis, spiritual care inside of lifestyle medicine, draws the person to transcendence and this "coherence," to what matters most to them. This is finding what will motivate them to extend themselves to meeting their own and other human needs while finding their own connection to transcendence, to the Force where they sense caring, to a Higher Power, to God. Spiritually sensitive care produces this life-centering effect which facilitates positive wellness even in the midst of pain and brokenness.

From another perspective, astronauts circling the Earth experienced this encounter with something greater than themselves, a new awareness and arrangement of self to the world called the "overview effect of awe and self-transcendence."[42] What they experienced was "a sacred encounter that entails a change in their vertical and or horizontal relationships,"[43] which means a change of self with the transcendent/ God and with other people. One very early childhood memory of this author is hearing Apollo 8 astronauts Frank Borman, Jim Lovell, and Bill Anders reading from Genesis on Christmas Eve. This author felt the overview effect herself while looking at Earth on television. If you are wondering about this, listen to the Apollo 8 astronauts and notice your own responses to their reactions (https://www.youtube.com/watch?v=njpWalYduU4). Remember, this broadcast followed them losing radio signal on the far side of the moon, the first time in history that humans were in orbit without radio signal.

For another metaphor for this sense of spirituality, consider the Japanese art form kintsugi. The artist takes pieces of broken ceramic pottery and mends them back together with gold, creating a unique and intricate work of art. The essence of this is that new beauty emerges from the old, often with renewed strength and resilience from the very places where the ceramic was broken apart. This occurs through the caring attentiveness of the artist applying the gold. Consider what comes together inside of you as you apply this metaphor to your nutrition practice and what your emotional availability can render in your client's life.

## Transcendence and meaning: *A path to a flourishing life?*

What's more, when clients and practitioners seek this positive wellness, are they just seeking more wellness to maximize the client's wellness and minimize suffering, or are they seeking to balance their lifestyle, harmonize their strengths with their weaknesses, and reconcile the good with the unavoidable bad? If we look to Oishi S, Westgate ED (2022), a significant number of people seek "a psychologically rich life which involves diverse and complex experiences and emotions, including sometimes negative feelings and experiences."[44] The writings of Victor Frankl seem to concur. Working through his trauma and suffering stemming from his time in the concentration camp during WWII, Frankl found a novel life perspective: "Healing comes through meaning"[45] from finding what holds life together, the integrating force of humans grounded in something greater, to the transcendence, in spite of the pain.

As you consider these thoughts, this whole chapter and Frankl's writing, let the words waft over you as you read them. Grasp what moves you:

 *When we are no longer able to change a situation, we are challenged to change ourselves. Everything can be taken from a man but one thing: the last of human freedoms — to choose one's attitude in any given set of circumstance, to choose one's way.*

Transformative learning can change us to find meaning and purpose in practicing dietetics or lifestyle medicine and in living flourishing lives. From your own growth, you become more able to nurture the same type of growth in clients, moving from just health to well-being practitioners who promote life flourishing. If nutritional professionals admit that sometimes they feel ill-equipped to handle highly emotional topics, they can choose to consider the thoughts that resonate with them and grow. Even though they may see health holistically, as wellness that integrates a good balance physically, emotionally, socially, and even spiritually, they may not know how to move beyond simply extending empathy and building rapport. With this in mind, however, you may still be wondering: how do I, as a dietitian or a lifestyle medicine provider, offer holistic care to address my client's spiritual issues while staying within the primary focus of my discipline?

While the remainder of this work will attempt to weave together a method for dietitians, nutritionists and healthcare providers to answer this question, we close this chapter with some thoughts from social psychologist David Meyer[46] to consider why we are attempting to bridge spiritual care and meaning-making with nutrition practice and health promotion. Consider his words and note for yourself any resonance, conflict, or motivation that stirs within you. He shared:

> *More than ever, we at the end of the last century were finding ourselves with big houses and broken homes, high incomes and low morale, secured rights and diminished civility. We were excelling at making a living but too often failing at making a life. We celebrated our prosperity but yearned for purpose. We cherished our freedoms but longed for connection.*
> *In an age of plenty, we were feeling spiritual hunger.*

Maybe these thoughts and the evidence that follows will assist you in seeing the client sitting before you in a new light and show how healthy eating and lifestyle can be best grounded in a life of well-being to create a community around you that is flourishing in body, mind, and spirit. In the question of Russo-Netzer (2023) can you become an agent of transformation who helps those you work with find "a sense of significance, worth and mattering?"[47] Listening for and incorporating your client's spirituality into nutrition care may just be the secret spice that can transform your practice from ordinary to the savory practice that encourages both you and the clients you work with to feed the hunger of the soul.

In summary, consider your own life, your traumas, difficulties, strengths, and limitations. We all have them. Consider what touches you in this reading and in what you are living right now. Make a commitment to seek what satisfies you, expands you, and brings you to positive wellness — what brings your life together. Many of your clients and even yourself, at times, seek to fill this golden place with food or striving. It's like they have been living on the far side of the moon.

# CHAPTER 2

*The Role of Spirituality in Dietetics*

*and Lifestyle Medicine*

Many within the field of nutrition and dietetics have been calling to incorporate holistic care into the nutrition care process for a number of years. Writing for the Academy, then the *Journal of the American Dietetic Association*, practitioners Annette Warpeha and Jeannette Harris (1993) emphasized that "wellness is a balance between body, mind, and spirit as a quest for harmony and inner peace."[48] These two innovative practitioners in private practice admonished dietitians "to look beyond balancing diet and exercise to encompass all aspects of what it means to be human; that is, living lives that are balanced emotionally, spiritually, physically, intellectually, and socially." They described their therapeutic approaches as "not typically associated with nutrition, but nevertheless those approaches that can help remove obstacles to behavioral change and enhance the outcome of a visit." Warpeha and Harris encouraged "a major shift in the use of therapeutic skills to combine traditional and nontraditional approaches to nutrition counseling through the use of meditation, guided imagery, therapeutic touch," and techniques commonly used in clinical chaplaincy, including "life reminiscence and the power of supportive presence." They asked patients to tell their stories. As practitioners leading the way to where we are now, Warpeha and Harris encouraged providers to grow affectively, writing, "When we are comfortable enough with another's pain or suffering that we can be there, then profound interactions can occur. Caring is healing."

When dietitians inquire into a patient's personal culture and existential questions, they successfully utilize the person's spirituality to motivate health behavior change. Dittman[49] et al. (2008) conducted a study with women (n-158) and explored spiritual beliefs, body awareness, body responsiveness, intuitive eating, body satisfaction, and spiritual readiness through questionnaires when they took part in postural yoga. They found that the women who cultivated spiritual readiness through the practice of mindfulness, developing spiritual beliefs while undertaking postural yoga, had greater improvements in body satisfaction, quality of life, eating attitudes, and disordered eating compared to the participants who undertook yoga alone with low spiritual readiness markers. With African American women, spiritual growth increased personal responsibility for health decisions, stress management, and promoted increased self-esteem and healthy eating and exercise behavior patterns. Spiritual growth supported this development when health promotion was offered at church or in social group settings.[50]

Dietitians, along with chaplains, designed the 7 Stepping Stone program at a VA hospital for 20 participants to promote diabetes self-management and weight loss, incorporating encouraging words and spiritual readings into the 7 key themes for diabetes self-management training (DSMT). The program, which was non-denominational from a Christian perspective, found that 55% of participants experienced increased personal coping, and 80% experienced significant behavior changes. The most common complaints about the 7 Stepping Stone program were that veterans sometimes felt confused between religion and spirituality and that the spiritual enrichment was Christian only in focus.[51] Spiritual growth and readiness that is encouraged using a variety of methods, in a variety of settings, according to the patient's culture and values, shows a positive impact on the acquisition of health behaviors and health metrics as well as wellness.

These thoughts are echoed in a provocative review by Morris et al. that suggests the need to utilize whole-person metrics in assessing renal patients' well-being, more than phosphate blood levels, to "capture the quality of the whole care provided, something that really matters to people who have kidney disease."[52] They suggest that personal well-being and health metrics can improve when practitioners offer empathetic and supportive care and take time to really get to know their patients and their "social, physical, spiritual, and emotional needs." These human aspects can impact dietary intake and need to be addressed in dietetic care, as poor follow-through with recommendations may stem from a lack of motivation due to feeling isolated and misunderstood. For many, spirituality and religion are key personal values.

## Today, are dietitians taking the initiative to speak about spirituality with their clients?

On the whole, dietitians see the profession as therapeutic, involving active listening by the practitioner as patients speak about their health in order to gather a deeper understanding of their needs. Gesser-Edelsburg describes this as "counseling about food and eating to find solutions for specific immediate problems," which arise from the "connection between body and soul."[53] Consider that maybe many dietitians all along have been delving into human/spiritual factors that lie beneath the science.

For example, in a one-to-one conversation that this author had with a spiritually astute dietitian, she described instinctively understanding this connection when she shared her experiences of going to a man's home for nutrition counseling while he was in end-stage renal disease. She said, "I think he wants to review his life and what has been important and impactful to him as he considers whether to continue with dialysis. I am going to give him space to speak about this because it seems really important to him, almost more than understanding the phosphorus levels of his foods."

This discussion is echoed in the work of Lycett,[54] who undertook a novel study to assess dietitians' perceptions (n=37) and practices in incorporating spiritual care into nutrition counseling/care. The results present a promising but mixed and complex picture. Utilizing a survey integrated from literature and questionnaires that had been used with other healthcare disciplines, this instrument was customized to be relevant to dietetics and given to dietitians who practiced in a variety of settings. Participants rated their responses using either a 5-point Likert scale or a 1–10 scale. Most showed a strong endorsement that religion/spirituality was important in its own right (3.9 out of 5 possible) and moderate support that it helped with everyday work (3.5 out of 5 possible). Dietitians seemed somewhat less convinced that spiritual care impacted physical health (3.5 out of 5 possible) or that religion/spirituality impacted patients' capacity to change eating behavior (3.6 out of 5 possible).

These same dietitians also seemed to question whether providing spiritual care was relevant to their practice, as evidenced by their ratings of the relevance for dietitians to assess spiritual needs (2.1 out of 5 possible), to facilitate patients' search for meaning in illness (2.8 out of 5 possible), and to support patients in gaining acceptance of their illness (3.3 out of 5 possible). In contrast, 92% utilized an assessment that addresses spiritual needs always or sometimes.

Dietitians from Lycett's 2024 study also showed a low response to the negative questioning, "I do not feel spiritual care is part of the dietitian's role" (2.2 out of 5 possible), which indicated that they felt that spiritual care was part of their role. This contrasts with how occupational therapists viewed spiritual care inside their discipline: "Less than 40% thought that spiritual care was part of their scope of practice."[55]

An interesting observation that Lycett (2024) sets forward from the current practice section is that "for some, the identification of the need for spiritual care was more in keeping with the role of the dietitian than with the delivery of spiritual care itself." If the patients raised spiritual issues, they attempted to "listen carefully (answering 4.6 out of 5 possible) and encourage service users in their own religious/spiritual practices (answering 4.0 out of 5 possible). These dietitians showed low confidence, however, in their ability to offer spiritual care (4.7 out of 10 possible) and voiced that they struggled to identify who had spiritual issues to discuss and how to deal with these issues once identified. They indicated that their "on-the-job training and academic training was inadequate to promote confidence in offering spiritual care (2.5 out of 5 and 1.9 out of 5, respectively). Probably in light of these feelings of insecurity about addressing spiritual needs, they showed a strong interest in more education in spiritual care (4.1 out of 5 possible) and displayed an openness to discussing spiritual needs/issues (4.1 out of 5).

The most common barriers to offering spiritual care were a lack of time, not having the right language to address the issues, or the worry that discussing spirituality would negatively impact their relationship with the patient or, for a minority of respondents, get them into trouble at work (Lycett, 2024). Overall, these findings seem to indicate that dietitians may not understand what is involved in offering spiritual assessment and spiritual care, how spirituality impacts physical health, body satisfaction, and overall well-being, or how it motivates human flourishing. The confusion appears to stem from a misunderstanding that spiritual care is more than praying with patients, using spiritual vocabulary, or knowing a Scripture to present to them, as few attempted to help patients find meaning in illness, assess for spiritual needs, or support their processing of end-of-life care.

These conclusions are reinforced by results from a study by Heyen (2021), who examined the impact of dietitians' intrinsic religiosity and continuing education on whether dietitians offered spiritual care to their patients. While a majority of the dietitians, 84%, felt that "sensitivity to clients' religious and spiritual beliefs will improve their practice," 80.3% rarely or never used empirically supported religious and spiritual interventions in their treatment."[56] These figures of Heyen mirror the results from occupational therapists, where 84% rated spirituality very important to health and rehabilitation but less than 40% "indicated that addressing clients' spiritual needs was within their scope of professional practice."[57]

However, in Heyen's work, 66.1% think they have not been adequately trained in spiritual care to offer this aspect to their clients. Similar to nurses, dietitians do appear more likely to offer this if they possess an intrinsic sense of their own spirituality or religion and have completed professional education on spiritual care.[58] With the occupational therapists, 82% of Engquist's (1997) sample thought that their academic training did not prepare them to work with their clients' spiritual needs. Lycett's (2024) results do not show that the dietitian's own religiosity had as strong an impact on their willingness to discuss spiritual needs. Her study participants were somewhat evenly split between religious (54%) and non-religious (46%), although a higher number rated themselves as spiritual (62%) compared to (38%). A majority indicated they would be open to discussing spiritual needs, answering 4.1 out of 5 for their willingness to discuss spiritual needs. Healthcare professionals appear open to delving into the spiritual aspects of living that could impact health, but across the board, they feel they need more training to be able to do so. A first step is to more fully understand spirituality, spiritual needs, spiritual distress, and grief.

# CHAPTER 3

*Understanding Spirituality and*

*Spiritual Needs in Lifestyle Medicine*

## What has been discussed about spirituality & being spiritually intelligent so far?

Understanding how to recognize positive spirituality is very helpful for nutrition and other healthcare professionals so they can notice it in themselves and the patients they serve. Cultivating this life-enhancing aspect of living can be part of what a dietitian includes in the assessment and plans, and monitors in follow-up sessions as a helpful dimension that promotes nutritional and physical health. Your clients' culture, religion, and spirituality impact how they hear and respond to the nutrition message that you send them and the goals they choose to manage their everyday activities. For example, a Buddhist client with excess weight seeking to reduce body weight may engage in the process more easily if it's couched as a means that improves posture for quiet centering meditation rather than a means of self-control. This is because spirituality is a positive force that usually helps motivate positive self-care and lifestyle behaviors. If the message is interpreted culturally for a client, they can best follow through with the guidance.

What you, as a provider, are after is to share ideas for self-care that are consistent with the client's culture and to develop a deeper understanding of how clients experience their spirituality. Many who have sought to define spirituality, however, have struggled to pin it down and have come up with the sense of it as "a uniting force in a divided and consumption-oriented world"[59] while others define it as a "connection with the Divine and awareness."[60] A growing trend is not to try to define it at all but to notice what it manifests and how each person reacts to it, their subjective experience of it, to know what is real. For some, the movement, too, is to step from an individually focused spirituality to a collective spirituality that aids society in more harmonious living.

If we admit it, this question of how to integrate spirituality into healthcare is a Western question when we compare our quest to countries in the East, where "spirituality is already far better integrated into health care... and research shows that this has clear positive effects."[61] Nita suggests that in healthcare in the East, spirituality is "not the silent dimensions or not overtly set in opposition to secularity and therefore is not pushed into the private sphere." In the West, to admit the questions and invite a discussion about grappling with spirituality is a counter-cultural movement. It acknowledges that science is not a stand-alone but another tool to integrate with our subjective experiences of spirituality.

What has been said so far is that spirituality is, in many ways, the golden glue that pulls life together: your experiences, both good and bad, with your values, motivations, and life energy. It helps you grow in existential intelligence and expand your living experience of the non-tangible but very real dynamics of spiritual connection to the sacred. This hopefully forms a coherence in life and assists you in experiencing greater meaning, purpose, creativity in living, and health or wellness, as well as connection with your Higher Power/Ultimate Reality.

According to Gordon Hilsman (2024), spirituality can also be described as the force that "ties together what a person cannot control, and that impacts the body, the psyche, sociability, and the soul."[62] It is the capacity to be moved by beauty, the beyond, as in the overview effect. The spiritual capacity can be a connection to something greater than ourselves, a transcendent one, to a Higher Power or to God, to a relationship with the Sacred, and to others with whom we live and serve.

It also has been inferred that spirituality grows when we slow down to notice, expose ourselves to beauty and creativity, and when we are attended to by others with support and warmth. This indicates that the spiritual flame can spark from one caring person to another. Remember hearing Taylor Swift and the community spirit at a concert with other "Swifters" or viewing Rembrandt, and how you may have felt inspired by their craft and moved affectively to be even more caring toward others. Using the work of Victor Frankl and *Man's Search for Meaning* (1963),[63] spirituality is more than just a feel-good sense; it is a force in living that brings forth grit and unflappability, as well as peace to the personality, and fosters resilience and persistence in doing good and living truthful, impactful lives.

## Some thoughts on spiritual care
## in the healthcare literature

The professions of nursing and occupational therapy have been exploring the integration of spiritual care into practice for a number of years, an observation based on a review of the literature from the last 45 years. Dietitians and lifestyle medicine professionals can find encouragement to incorporate spirituality into practice from the nursing profession as well as from occupational therapy,[64] along with some initial ideas from pharmacy.[65]

Dietitians, however, offer a unique aspect when spiritual care is integrated into practice, distinct from other disciplines, according to the reflections of this author. Spiritual care offers support beyond a focus on addressing "spiritual concerns" or problems, as is often focused upon in nursing (UKCC 1984 Code of Professional Conduct).[66] Typically, dietitians have longer sessions with clients, frequently emphasizing lifestyle factors that promote wellness and can effectively consider how spiritual/religious resources serve as health assets that draw the client to greater vitality and well-balanced living.

Today, the literature shows that nurses and occupational therapists both readily admit that spirituality is an important part of wellness and healthy living.[67] Nearly 60% of pharmacists agreed that religion and spirituality would likely be helpful to them if they were ill and would be helpful to know about a patient, but 96% of pharmacists surveyed had never talked with a patient about their spiritual or religious needs.[68]

Nurses are "generally willing to offer spiritual care to their patients"[69] but like many dietitians and lifestyle medicine providers, fail to follow through with this due to "lack of time" and "a feeling that they have not received adequate training" to offer multi-dimensional spiritual care while staying inside their discipline.[70] Meyer et al. also point out that the main reason nurses do not offer spiritual care is the lack of the nurses' own "level of religious commitment" or the lack of emphasis that was placed on spirituality in their nursing training.[71] Harrad (2019) further notes that the best modality for providing this training, in fact, was continuing professional development, which did promote "a willingness to guide patients to find inner peace (a specific facet of spiritual care)." Understanding that attending to spirituality can impact health and fit into a professional's ongoing assessment grows from an awareness of the spiritual dimension that the professional has started to recognize in their own life experience.

Speaking to nurses, Kytoko (1999) outlines the distinction between religion and spirituality, which often can confuse practitioners about where to start with holistic care. The two are distinct, yet "can overlap, relate to each other or exist separately."[72] Spirituality has been defined as a "dynamic principle or an aspect of the person that is related to God or gods, other people or aspects of personal being, or material nature,"[73] or the "unique array of ways that a person deals with the uncontrollable."[74]

Religion is a way spirituality can be lived but not every spiritual person is religious."[75] What's more, religion is "a set of beliefs, practices and language that characterizes a community that is searching for transcendent meaning in a particular way, generally based upon belief in a deity."[76] Members of a religion learn how to define themselves by "collective learning" and often see lifestyle behaviors modeled by each other.[77] An example of this is for the Muslim to wear a hijab as a head covering, to fast at Ramadan and to avoid smoking or alcohol as a means of praising God.

In many ways, in fact, religion can make processing spiritual issues and questions easier by "providing a community of faith and support and a readymade language with which to describe spiritual struggles and joys."[78] It can also give a healthcare provider a place to start their personal investigation into spirituality by providing sacred texts and spiritual practices.

- Baldacchino (2015) concurs in describing that spirituality "goes beyond religious affiliation, and is a human pursuit, as the spirit is that part of the person who finds fulfillment in life, suffering/death, and in hope for one's will to live."[79] She, along with Burnard, 1990 describes spirituality as striving for meaning and purpose, for inspiration in living, even for those who don't believe in God or a Higher Power, at least not yet.[80] Likewise, Narayanasamy (1999), a pioneer in spiritual care within nursing, said that spirituality is "part of the biological make-up of the human species and present in all individuals because of spirituality's biological survival value." It may manifest as "inner peace, strength derived from a perceived relationship with an Ultimate Reality or whatever an individual values as supreme."[81]

An expanded list from nursing literature, in fact, defines spirituality in a number of ways such as:

- The essence or life principle of the person (Colliton, 1981)[82]
- A Sacred Journey (Mische, 1982)[83]
- The experience of the radical truth of things (Legere, 1984)[84]
- Giving meaning and purpose in life, a life relationship or a sense of connection with mystery, a Higher Power, God or the Universe (Bradshaw, 1994[85] Granstrom, 1985)[86]
- A belief that relates a person to the world (Soeken and Carson, 1987)[87]

- A universal phenomenon, and that all of us possess and the spiritual dimension evokes feelings that demonstrate the existence of love, faith, hope, trust, awe and inspirations[88]
- "A search for the sacred or transcendent, a personal vertical relationship one establishes with what one deems sacred" (Teixeira Pinto, 2024).
- While this list and discussion may seem tedious or lengthy, having a variety of ways to recognize spirituality and understanding how it sometimes can differ from religiosity often helps non-chaplain healthcare providers identify a spiritual issue in the life and narrative of their patients.

## Learning from addiction recovery

Recovery programs for addictions successfully show how spirituality, spiritual assessment, and spiritual care can be integrated into an integrative treatment model. The addiction recovery process has successfully brought spiritual care into treatment and peer support for over 100 years. Twelve-step programs illustrate the aspects of spirituality listed above in action. Consider the Twelve Steps of AA, which many treatment centers use as a foundation to build their programs on, although not all do. In Step 1, a drunk or addict acknowledges that their life, as they know it right now, is unmanageable (no sense of coherence/meaning), and Step 2 brings forward the belief that a power greater than themselves—a Higher Power or a new awareness of transcendence—can restore them to sanity. Step 3 is their decision to turn their life over to this power because they have reached what seems like their human limits, so they can experience freedom and new life, a spiritual awakening. (Remember Victor Frankl's words: the most basic freedom that humans possess is the capacity to direct their choices, focus, and attitudes.)

Kurtz (1990)[89] describes that addicts find meaning by telling their stories in order to feel safe and connected to others so they can experience new life (an example of the power of a collective spirituality). He also speaks of a "letting go or a freedom that allows them to escape from the savage mastery of the addiction." He further elucidates the importance of getting in touch with "the hole at the center or core that addicts are using the addiction to fill."[90] This metaphor of the hole at the core suggests that there is something missing: a loss of purpose and love, a loss of a positive sense of self (lack of coherence or the framework or philosophy of Maslow), or a relationship with the divine, which centers, draws, and holds the fragile parts of the person together. Without this sense of purpose, addicts experience the sense of "spiritual hunger" described earlier and, prior to treatment, use the addiction to slacken.

Do clients welcome this emphasis on spirituality in treatment centers? DiReda and Gonsalvez (2016)[91] describe that "94% of study participants, addicts in residential treatment, desire and welcome a spiritual focus in their care." DiReda also notes that "if addicts do not include an awareness and focus on spirituality and don't integrate it into the treatment," the maintenance of healthy behaviors is short-lived. They describe spirituality as the glue or cohesion that holds abstinence (a healthy lifestyle) together against discombobulating forces: the isolation, disconnect, and emotional traumas that come from addiction.

As addictions cut across the board and impact people from all cultural backgrounds, and considering the interesting sense that spirituality itself is a universal human need and attribute as described earlier, the words of Sulmasy provide support for this and helpful insights for understanding the importance of addressing spiritual concerns. Including spirituality and spiritual care in treatment appears to meet basic human needs. He states, "I am fully persuaded that as a Christian speaks out of the fullness of Christian conviction, and a Buddhist speaks out of the fullness of Buddhist conviction, and the atheist speaks out of the fullness of atheist conviction, deep spiritual resonance will occur and each can learn enormously from the others."[92] For lifestyle medicine, helping a client tap into their spirituality, life coherence or spiritual resonance is tremendously healing for the person, body, mind, and soul.

## How faith or "the quest for meaning" matures

Before an exploration of spirituality closes, a few words are necessary to discuss the developmental nature of spirituality, faith, and sense of meaning. Experience, perception, and expression of faith are not static but grow along with a person's human faculties: their abilities to perceive, emote, and understand life, according to Fowler (1981).[93] Some have considered this life-span developmental process as "Multidirectional, adaptive and involving gains and losses,"[94] one that follows distinct stages of growth. It seems easier to describe this by comparing spiritual growth to

Kohlberg's model of moral development[95] or Piaget's Cognitive Development Stages. The direction in which faith grows is from the concrete to the more abstract, from a focus principally on the individual and their own holiness to a focus on community and the greater good of a wider circle. Spirituality and religion grow from strong reliance on the precepts of authority to greater reliance on one's own perceptions and personal ownership/agency, from absolutes to a greater sense of mystery.

This can impact the practitioner who is charged with understanding the perspectives of others from different traditions, a task that may be very difficult if the clinician has a strongly defended faith or is less flexible in finding value in other perspectives or has a narrower perception or "social horizons" where faith differences are harder to value. This awareness can also help caregivers recognize faith more easily if they are aware that it can be voiced with different nuances. A person with a more mature faith or sense of spirituality carries along with these aspects of earlier phases of faith development. For example, they can value the teachings from authorities and be moved by beliefs and the witness of their faith community to more mystical spiritual practices. They may have a strong sense of right and wrong and follow God and the needs of social order, but they live this awareness with more mystery and universal values that draw them from within.

While there are accounts of several young children who were mystics and moved by the plight of the world, when a practitioner is working with pediatric or adolescent patients and with some adults who remain concrete, rule-bound thinkers, they may find it best to listen for how they live these concrete beliefs and use concrete symbols or sacred texts from the patient's tradition to help the client tap into their spirituality as a resource for their health. These people may worry about rules and rubrics, and suggesting yoga, meditation, etc., may bring undue anxiety, whereas having them recite a familiar prayer as a mind/body/spiritual practice will not.

Faith/spirituality is a force that can bring stability and is designed in ever-expanding ways to assist a person to "make sense of their experiences, detect patterns and establish a sense of predictability in the world."[96]

## Does religion impact the goals clients set, and what motivates in nutrition education or lifestyle medicine?

With increasing immigration in many areas of the world, understanding cultures different from your own and the impact of religion on health behaviors and goals becomes very important. For example, as a practitioner considers helping a client formulate a SMART goal, besides making it specific, measurable, and obtainable, it needs to fit with the client's cultural and religious priorities. According to McCullough & Willoughby (2009),[97] spirituality and religion influence goal selection. As a case in point, Christians, both Catholic and Protestant, and Jews more often pursue goals that offer higher-arousal emotional states that instill excitement, enthusiasm, and euphoria, which move and reinforce their actions. On the other hand, in the words of McCullough & Willoughby, Buddhists more often value low-arousal affective states and work more toward goals that promote calm, peacefulness, or relaxation. Cultural norms influence priorities.

It is also noted in support of this that "Christian religious texts place a higher value on high arousal positive affective states and a lower value on low arousal positive affective states than do Buddhist religious texts."[98] So, lifestyle goals, such as encouraging a Buddhist client to increase morning light or to consume chamomile tea to calm them, may be appropriate, while for Christians and Jews, focusing on eating more healthy foods, like fats or carbohydrates for energy, may be more appropriate.

In a systematic review of religion, self-regulation, and self-control, McCullough & Willoughby showed that personal religiosity and behavioral self-control were significantly related. They posited that religiosity regulated the selection of appropriate goals and motivated goal-seeking, even sanctifying certain goals involving self-regulation (i.e., fasting during Ramadan or Lent). Likewise, high levels of religiosity promoted personality traits of conscientiousness that encouraged "higher levels of physical activity, less alcohol, tobacco and drug use, healthier eating habits, safer driving." Health providers who follow the lead of patients, listen attentively to their narratives and practices, and suggest or reflect a goal that correlates with the client's spirituality can aid compliance and follow-through.

Results from Azari NP, Missimer & Seitz (2005)[99] also showed that study participants who were experienced with meditative prayer likewise showed weaker anterior cortical responses (measured by ECG) to aversive messages compared to those who did not pray. This means that they experienced a greater willingness to follow through with what they heard in the health message. Also, the experienced praying participants, as they prayed during the MRI, showed an "increase in activity in the prefrontal cortex, areas promoting executive function, attention, conflict monitoring, and cognitive control."[100] These changes in executive function could promote better self-management and follow-through. In this light, when someone comes to a session with low energy, the clinician may assist the patient in engaging with the session by suggesting a moment of quiet reflection in order to activate their brain for the session.

Another interesting aspect is how Christians and Jews tend to differ in how they work with thoughts of actions. According to Cohen (2003),[101] Christians can "violate religious principles just by thinking and entertaining a negative thought like "lust, violent thoughts, contemplating the commission of a dishonest act." Jews, on the other hand, according to Cohen (2003), "believe that thoughts in and of themselves are neither blameworthy nor praiseworthy which means that Protestant and Catholic Christians may set goals about controlling their thoughts, that religious Jews evidently do not." Likewise, Muslims see religion as a lifestyle with outside manifestations, whereas in Europe (and the United States), religion is more a private matter that is not so often exposed.[102] Consider too, for example, the possible spiritual distress of a Christian client who obsesses over their weight, food or binge-eating behavior. Practitioners may misunderstand and sidetrack clients if they misread the cultural and religious dynamics.

"Patients require healthcare professionals to understand their wider cultural and spiritual needs when providing healthcare advice."[103] Religion often promotes certain ways of doing ordinary things, such as Hindus using different hands for eating and toileting, obeying dietary laws, following regulations for food preparation, and ritually fasting on specific days.[104] These values also "influence the understanding of illness, health-seeking behavior and medical compliance."[105] For Muslims, eating healthy foods, formulating healthy routines/practices and fasting during the month of Ramadan are seen as a religious duty and a way of praising God.[106]

This change in a person's capacity to manage their choices and practice self-management and control may also be facilitated by the effect of religiosity/spirituality and sense of purpose on the brain. Similar to the previous study mentioned, Kang et al. (2020)[107] took 220 sedentary adults and monitored activity in the brain structures associated with regulating conflicts via MRI while participants heard messages to increase their physical activity. Those who scored high in meaning and purpose after filling out a seven-question questionnaire also showed significantly less arousal or activity in the conflict centers of the brain than those who heard the same message but rated themselves as less spiritual. This indicates that when patients experience less activity in the conflict centers, they may experience less resistance or conflict in receiving a health promotion message, which could make follow-through easier.

Moving from an understanding of how spirituality can surface in life and be described in a patient interaction is only part of the learning process. Each practitioner needs to consider and describe their own spirituality to apply what they learned. Fill out the following spirituality reflection and spiritual checklist and reflect with your answers.

# Describe your Spirituality:
## Check all that apply

☐ Way to find meaning/purpose

☐ Way to cope with suffering, death, Find joy, hope, faith or love

☐ The essence or life principle of a person

☐ Part of human biological make-up

☐ Manifests peace, strength, resiliency

☐ A relationship with God, Higher Power or the Sacred

☐ A Sacred Journey

☐ The experience of radical truth

☐ A belief that relates a person to the world

☐ A universal phenomenon. All people possess

☐ A search for the sacred or transcendent in living

☐ A personal vertical relationship with God or higher Power

## Questions to consider:

Does my life feel out of control or overwhelming sometime?

Do I sense a power greater than myself that I can turn to?

How would I describe that central theme or sense of coherence in my life?

How do I cultivate a connection to What I experience as Sacred?

## My clarity statement:

Write a statement that clarifies your own spiritual perspectives

**My Answers to the questions to consider:**

**My clarity statement How do I describe my spirituality**

# Spirituality Reflection

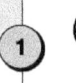

### Reflect with spirituality, what resonates

To grow and clarify your thoughts on spirituality, there are three steps: action, reflection and action. Read over the checklist on the next page, reflect and check off aspects of your own spiritual values.

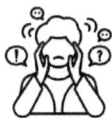

### Does my life feel out of control?

Serving others as a healthcare professional involves admitting your own vulnerability. Consider if your life feels out of control or stressed sometime. Do you sense a central theme or coherence that grounds your life?

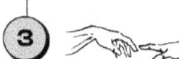

### Do I find a power greater than self?

As you live, do you sense a power greater than yourself that you can turn to when you experience your limits? How would you describe this power, force or goodness that surrounds you?

### Do I cultivate a connection to Sacred?

From your own experiences, how do you cultivate a connection to the sacred? Is it in nature, in intimate conversation, in prayer or in reading sacred texts/rituals?

### My questions and clarity statement

From this exercise, answer the questions on the next page and write out your own clarity, spiritual or statement of faith that describes your own spirituality.

# CHAPTER 4

*Is there Evidence that Positive*

*Spirituality Promotes Physical Health*

*and Personal WellBeing?*

Let us explore the evidence that positive spirituality and religious coping make a real difference in physical health, personal well-being, and all-cause mortality. While this information may seem tedious, this author has learned that lifestyle practitioners and especially Registered Dietitians, need to see the evidence that spiritual issues impact health. To start, we examine a large study (Boylan et al., 2023) that investigated the impact of religious and spiritual identity, coping, and spirituality on all-cause mortality in the Midlife in the United States (MIDUS) study, n=6120. Boylan et al. found that "religious and spiritual coping, spirituality, and religious identification were collectively and independently associated with lower mortality risks over a 25-year follow-up (1995–2020)."[108] A one standard deviation increase in these religious/spiritual variables produced a 6–9% decrease in the hazard rate after adjusting for age, sex, race, marital status, education, and chronic health conditions. The results showed that this effect on all-cause mortality was mediated by two factors: having a stronger sense of meaning/purpose in living and more positive relations with others. In fact, positive religious and spiritual coping comes, when a person has a secure relationship with a transcendent force and uses this relationship to cope with challenges. This leads "to greater purpose in living, which is positively related to better lifestyle behaviors."[109] The positive collective sense that comes with being connected to others pursuing a similar life purpose also appears to correlate with a lower mortality rate in living. Positive spirituality makes a significant impact on longevity and physical well-being.

Using data from the MIDUS2 study (n = 2,060 from the USA, 57.5% normal weight, 75% college educated), the 10-year longitudinal follow-up to the initial phase of the 25-year study, Berkowitz expanded earlier findings. He also utilized data from the CHILEMED interventional study (Clinical Trials NCT05454906) carried out between 2021 and 2024, examining the impact of healthy eating and psychological well-being in reversing metabolic syndrome in 330 Chilean participants with metabolic syndrome (ages 25 to 70 years old, 75% were college educated, and less than 5% normal weight). Earlier findings showed that a stronger purpose in living was correlated with greater consumption of vegetables and/or fruits.[110] Berkowitz found that for both groups, the USA group and the Chilean cohort, a higher purpose in living was associated with higher scores on the healthy eating index (healthy eating for the culture and low-fat dietary patterns). Likewise, a higher sense of meaning and purpose was consistently associated with a smaller waist circumference, an indicator of abdominal obesity, most likely produced by healthier food intake. The CHILEMED and MIDUS2 results support the idea that a high sense of purpose in life may bring about better health and reduce the risk of non-communicable metabolic illness by decreasing abdominal obesity, which is mediated through "protective/restorative behaviors: healthy eating."[111] Clearly, growing spiritually produced very helpful effects on metabolism by motivating health-promoting behaviors.

Greater spiritual and religious coping which impacted meaning and purpose were correlated with the ability to make and develop healthier food choices and habits which appeared to enhance bodily function by reducing inflammatory markers (Morozink et al., 2010[112], Cole et al., 2015[113], Guimond et al., 2022[114]). This was especially noted in men according to Guimond & Shiba (2022),[115] which found that the protective effect of meaning and purpose "lowered the hazard of developing unhealthy CRP. For all participants, both men and women,however, higher purpose in living correlated with a slower rise in CRP over time that is associated with aging." These findings are in step with Dalmida et al. (2011),[116] who also found that women with HIV/AIDS with higher scores on existential well-being had lower CD4 cell counts, and lower HIV viral loads. Positive spirituality is anti-inflammatory as it lowers levels of inflammation in the body.

In like fashion, there is increasing evidence that spiritual practices like meditation, quiet focusing/prayer, and mindfulness—a practice of focusing attention in the moment of daily life—are associated with significant benefits that reduce inflammation and promote more optimal methylation of DNA, silencing genes that promote inflammation. In a small study by Chaix et al., 2020),[117] 17 participants with experience of meditation and 17 participants with similar patterns of DNA methylation but with no experience of meditation went on a one-day experience. The participants with prayer experience meditated for a one-day period (8 hours), while the controls had a day of leisure activities. The meditators activated 61 different methylation sites that effectively silenced or turned off genes promoting inflammation, positively regulated immune cell metabolism associated with cell-mediated immunity and aging, and reduced binding sites for several transcription factors involved in immune response and inflammation. The control group showed no increases in the activation of methylation binding sites, so they were more prone to inflammation and aging.

Likewise, results of Kaliman et al. (2014)[118] found that a similar group of participants meditating intensively for one day (n=19), as compared to matched participants (n=21) undertaking leisure activities without meditation, showed a significant decrease in the expression of pro-inflammatory genes (RIPK2 and COX2) and a reduction in histone deacetylase genes (HDAC2,3 and 9) which have been implicated in decreased neuronal plasticity, cognitive decline and Alzheimer's Disease. Meditation appeared to make the nervous system more plastic or flexible.

Religious coping and greater spiritual intelligence also decrease inflammation and positively impact many other chronic diseases, which becomes even clearer. Positive spirituality has been associated with better glucoregulation,[119] according to Rasmussen et al. 2013,[120] along with others,[121] a reduced risk of cardiovascular disease,[122] and less cognitive degeneration.[123] Researchers also have noted that spirituality is negatively correlated with symptoms of depression from the work of Bamonti (2016),[124] indicating that spirituality impacts many aspects of mental health as well as physical disease via impacting inflammation. When spirituality is clearly shown to decrease inflammation, it behooves dietitians and other healthcare professionals to incorporate spiritual care principles into lifestyle and nutrition care practices and to grow in spiritual intelligence themselves.

These results seem to concur with Fox (1994),[125] who said that human beings possess both an inner life as well as an outer life and that nourishing attention to the inner life can lead to a more meaningful and engaging outer life. The relationship between spirituality, health behaviors, and psychological health was elucidated by Bozek et al. 2020,[126] who noted that although both spirituality and healthy behaviors strengthened psychological well-being, "spirituality is, in fact, a determinant of psychological well-being prior to health-related behaviors." With this in mind, clinicians can step forward to not just notice spiritual issues but also take an active role in helping clients meet their spiritual needs, which builds both psychological health and strengthens resolve for health-related behaviors.

High levels of positive spirituality in a person's life have been shown to change their perception of life and capacity to manage choices and follow through with health behaviors. For example, in patients with type 2 diabetes, high levels of spiritual development activated patient responsibility for self-care, leading to increased self-efficacy regarding dietary planning and the type and quantity of food consumed, as noted by Duke (2021),[127] although not for exercise.

## Spirituality's impact on relationship with the body

Spirituality also predicts better appreciation of the body and quality of life measures.[128] Older men who experience intrinsic religiosity (internalized religious beliefs that they seek to live) indicate a stable, warm relationship with God; an overall sense of satisfaction, meaning, and purpose in life; and see their bodies as a manifestation and expression of God are also more satisfied with their bodies. For older women, higher body satisfaction was only weakly associated with church attendance, intrinsic religious beliefs, and overall positive satisfaction with their lives).[129] Homan proposes that women associate body image with their faith differently than men, as women showed less body anxiety at older ages after having struggled more often with poor body image in their younger years and, over the years, having turned more often to their spirituality for solace. This movement for older men to now connect body image to their faith for comfort shows that "body dissatisfaction was substantially higher for men, and religion seems to have a positive role in maintaining whatever body satisfaction they have."

When presented with an unknown or a challenge, such as aging or, in this case, a diagnosis of cancer, spiritually oriented patients were able to view their vulnerabilities differently in a way that promoted personal growth. For example, coping with adversity, according to Penman (2021),[130] "precipitates transformation affecting the identity, sense of self, thinking processes, replacing negative thoughts with positive ones, relationships and behaviors." Macquarrie (1972)[131] describes that those changes in health, wellness needs, or even during serious illness draw a person toward their core or something greater when they "face emotional stress, physical illness or death." When a person experiences these changes, they experience personal vulnerability and begin to ask different questions, which can catalyze new openness to growth/change and lifestyle medicine. This growth seems to support the positive impact of intrinsic faith, as it provides solace and perspective in the face of the unknown and a capacity for a person to utilize their psychological resources.

In order to get comfortable navigating often emotionally charged topics—a client's spirituality, distress, and what gives them meaning and purpose—you need to become more aware of your own feelings, needs, and unexplored reactions that can impact how available you are to these challenges in others. I am remembering an emergent call I had to attend, a young couple who had just experienced the stillbirth of their baby. The deceased infant, dressed in a crochet outfit, lay in the mother's arms. As I walked in, I felt tears well up in my eyes. This was five years after I had also lost a baby through miscarriage. By staying aware of my own pain points, I was able to move my own experiences from front and center to the side somewhat and attend to supporting this couple. In the course of our interaction, I allowed the tears to fall gently on my face. We were welcoming the reality together, and in that, I think they felt supported and the power of compassion. Without having worked with the transformative learning process similar to what the second portion of this book describes, I fear I may have been unable to remain available to them.

What you are reviewing in the next section is a verbatim or direct verbal replay of a counseling session, along with the practitioner's feelings and flow of thoughts that give clues to the practitioner's own inner landscape. Self-reflection can help a professional grow and address their emotional and spiritual needs, impacting their care for others. This verbatim is meant to illustrate how spiritual care flows naturally within nutrition counseling.

Review this verbatim to follow the flow of the session and how spiritual themes arose, the feelings voiced, and the reactions of the practitioner. How does this dietitian bring spirituality into the session? Would you do anything differently? What feelings surface for you as you observe this interplay?

# An example of spiritual care (SC) inside of nutrition counseling:
## The Verbatim Report 1

## I. INFORMATION about the Client:

Middle-aged postmenopausal woman who had met with me for three sessions prior to this session and stopped because she thought that she could handle managing her eating behavior herself. She initiated today's session for ongoing support because she had seen her weight creeping up 8 pounds in 6 weeks. She denies any symptoms of edema. She has pre-diabetes, hypertension and is 50 lbs above her typical adult weight of 150 lbs. at 63 inches height. Her weight has gradually been going up since menopause. She has a consistent pattern of dieting through low-calorie, high-protein routines that she could not sustain. She struggles with worry about not feeling full enough and has emotional struggles eating with her husband at evening meal. She immigrated from South America at age 16. She works four 10-hour days at a human service position, a job she enjoys. This visit took place via Telehealth where she met with me from home on her day off. This was our fourth visit. We met for 45 minutes.

## II. OBSERVATIONS

What are your feelings going into the encounter? I felt happy to be visiting with her and curious about what she was experiencing.

What do you observe about the setting, the person, or the loved ones (e.g., notable contents or condition of the room, posture and gestures, mannerisms, clothing, etc.)? She appeared open to the engagement, as she spoke easily about her experiences and feelings. She appeared relieved to be speaking with me and spoke close to the camera.

## III. VERBATIM:  P = Provider, CL = Client

Record the visit as you recall it. Include any important non-verbal cues in parenthesis, your inner impressions and your inner dialogue and feelings.

Example: Try to remember as clear as you can the actual dialogue between you and the client that you want to process. Also note your own feelings and reactions while you worked with the client. Be as honest as you can so you can learn about yourself as you provide care.

P1: It's good to see you. Good to have a chance to speak. How are things going? *I felt happy to be speaking with her, as I cared about her and wondered what we would discuss to be helpful for her.*

CL1: Well, I'm really glad to speak with you. Since we talked last, my weight has gone up about eight pounds. I am so disgusted that I don't even want to get on the scale.

P2: That sounds really difficult. Can you tell me more about what's been going on?

CL2: Well, I struggle with having something cold foods to take for breakfast when I'm working, as we don't have a microwave in my work area. I still tried to take a protein, like boiled eggs, but I'm not wanting to get hungry, so I take carb foods to eat too, probably too much carb. I'm often really full after breakfast. Like I eat a large fruit and ½ of bagel with cream cheese with two boiled eggs. I find that I don't get hungry even at lunch but I eat lunch anyway. I usually take leftovers for lunch. (She showed me her carry-out container with veggies and rice in it.) Dinner is really difficult.

**P3: What's difficult about dinner?**

CL3: Well, you know the situation with my husband, he pressures me to eat with him in the evening even when I'm telling him that I'm not hungry. He often wants to eat foods like pizza, French fries, Hamburger Helper that don't appeal to me. I cook but I really don't feel hungry for these. He gets angry that I don't want to eat with him so I cave in and eat far more than I want to just to stop him. *I feel curious about what her husband is needing from her and where this interaction comes from.*

P4: How do you respond when he gets upset with you about not joining in eating the foods you made for him? *I felt compassion for her, as she has reported this interaction before.*

CL5: I stand my ground and tell him that I don't feel hungry and that he knows that these are not foods that I like, that I make them for him. This is nothing new. This interaction has been happening for a long time.

P5: So when you prepare the foods he likes and then don't join in with him in a meal to eat them, he gets angry with you or confronts you? *I feel perplexed about this interaction.*

CL6: Yes, I stand up to him but it really flusters me. I get all upset that he's pressuring me to eat. *I feel perplexed about the fact that even though she verbally states her position, eventually she gives in and overeats.*

P6: So even though you tell him you don't enjoy those foods and are not hungry, you do eat the foods?

CL7: Yes, And I get so disgusted with him and with myself. I say, well might as well eat and get him off my back. Then I look in the mirror and see my body so big. I have never been trying to be skinny but I really don't like my weight. When I plan a meal for myself, I really don't want to be hungry but I'm not sure how to portion things.

P7: So when he challenges you, you try to stand up for yourself but you eventually give in and then you don't eat in a way that feels good to you. You feel anger towards him, yourself or what?

CL8: Yes, I guess I do feel anger towards him and towards myself? *I feel compassion towards her and some frustration towards her husband. I am wondering if her need for autonomy is being touched on here?*

P8: So, when he confronts you, you get angry, speak back to defend yourself and then give in and eat and feel angry at yourself?

CL9: Yes. *She sat for a few minutes.* I never saw things like this. *She pauses and sits a moment.*

P9: And, when he challenges you, it hits on your autonomy? He's challenging your ability to have your say?

CL10: Yes, that is what's happening. She looked relieved.

P10: And when that need for autonomy gets touched on, you react. I wonder what he is needing in confronting you about not eating with him. Does that equal affirmation to him, or comradery? I wonder?

CL11: I don't know. I never had the clarity to consider what he was needing. I will pay attention this week to my reactions and what I notice about the interaction and how I overeat in response to this. I just really feel dislike about how I look in the mirror. *I noticed how she returned to her sense of body dissatisfaction.*

P11: So, eating and this struggle to have your voice brings you to also notice a dissatisfaction with your body and how you look?

CL12: Yes, I guess that's right, it all is kind of connected isn't it. I'm just so frustrated that I can't find the power to turn this around. *I wondered about her spirituality, as this can offer some power to turn this frustration around?*

P12: You'd like to find some power to feel differently and eat differently? Can you tell me about your spirituality? *I felt curious what would come from this question and hopeful it would help ground her in a new efficacy. Was this good timing?*

CL13: I'm a believer, a Christian. I see my body as a Temple of God and I want to know how to take care of it. I don't feel I have been taking care of it with this weight and blood sugar coming up.

P13: Is that something you'd like to connect with, with God?

CL14: Yes, and I know that God sees me in love. That would probably help me with this sense of not liking myself, and with getting so angry with my husband.

P14: Would you want to use a meditation: Loving Kindness Nourishment reflection? You could consider that God is with you in the reflection and see how that goes?

CL15: That sounds good. I'm going to write out 3 meals menus from the meal plan structure you gave me before and that Loving Kindness reflection sounds really nice. I will pay attention and consider what is going also on inside my husband. Thanks, this has really been helpful.

## V. EVALUATION & SUPERVISION

Why did you choose this nutrition counseling encounter? I chose this encounter because I saw several dimensions discussed that could be supported by spirituality. She was having struggles self-regulating with portions, most likely as a response to food restriction from previous diet attempts. She also was struggling to have a voice, and follow through in respect of her own wishes. She also was struggling with some body dissatisfaction.

What are you learning as you record this encounter? I am noticing how spirituality can play a part in the cohesion of self-care principles and in self-healing.

What do you learn about human nature, spirituality, and the Sacred in this encounter? As a dietitian, I helped her connect her values/faith to her struggle with lifestyle management, as well as provide her with non-partisan support. By including spirituality, she seemed to feel supported as a person.

What social or cultural forces are at work? I am unaware what cultural forces with men/women interactions might be at play, as she was from South America. I may bring this question forward in later sessions.

Where do you want supervision? How did spirituality support the movement of the session? Did I seem to stay with her in her emotional struggles rather than move her with my reactions?

## Example 1 of a spiritual assessment tool

What follows is a written spiritual assessment for you to use with yourself. The purpose is to get you thinking and recognizing ways your spirituality is bubbling up in your experience. When you learn to recognize subtle touches in your own life, you will be better able to recognize your clients' spiritual experiences and needs. A spiritual assessment can also provide a frame of reference for listening to patients and help you identify spiritual dimensions in their life stories and experiences. During this time, you may find it helpful to keep a journal of your spiritual moments and questions.

## The INSPIRIT Spiritual Assessment[132]

The following questionnaire will help you determine the degree to which you have developed your own personally meaningful spirituality. This can allow us to experience transformative growth and assist us to grow more resilient ourselves and more connected to others.

1. **How strongly religious or spiritually oriented do you consider yourself to be?**

   1. Not at all

   2. Not very strong

   3. Somewhat strong

   4. Strong

2. **About how often do you spend time on religious or spiritual practices?**

   Once per year or less

   Once per month to several times per year

   Once per week to several times per month

   Several times per day to several times per week

3. **How often have you felt as though you were very close to a powerful spiritual force?**

   Never

   Once or twice

   Several times

   Often

   People have many different images and definitions of the Higher Power we often call God. Use your image and your definition of God when answering the following questions.

4. **How close do you feel to God?**

   I don't believe in God

   Not very close

   Somewhat close

   Extremely close

5. **Have you ever had an experience that has convinced you that God exists?**

   No

   I don't know

   Maybe

   Yes

6. **Indicate whether you agree or disagree with this statement: "God dwells within you."**

   Definitely disagree

   Tend to disagree

   Tend to agree

   Definitely agree

7. The following list describes spiritual experiences that some people have had. Indicate if you have had any of these experiences and the extent to which each has affected your belief in God/HP. (1=Never had this experience, 2=Did not strengthen belief in God, 3=Strengthened belief in God, 4=Convinced me of God's Existence.

A. An experience of profound inner peace 1 2 3 4

B. An overwhelming experience of love 1 2 3 4

C. A feeling of unity with the earth and  all living beings 1 2 3 4

D. An experience of complete joy and ecstasy 1 2 3 4

E. Meeting or listening to a spiritual master or teacher 1 2 3 4

F. An experience of God's energy or presence 1 2 3 4

G. An experience of a great spiritual figure (Jesus, Mary, Elijah, Buddha) 1 2 3 4

H. A healing of your body or mind (or witnessed such a healing) 1 2 3 4

I. A miraculous (or not normally occurring) event 1 2 3 4

J. An experience of angels or guiding spirits 1 2 3 4

K. An experience of communication with someone who has died 1 2 3 4

L. An experience with near death or life after death 1 2 3 4

M. Other (Specify)

_____

_____

_____

_____

_____

_____

Add up your scores for questions 1–6. Your score should be between 6 and 24.

Question 7: Take the highest score for any question in 7 and add that to your first sum from questions 1–6. This is your score for the INSPIRIT.

Scoring: High Score = 25–28, Medium High = 18–24, Medium Low = 11–17, Low = 7–10

If your score is low, you may seek to explore your spirituality in a way consistent with your culture and experiences. If your score is high, it will confirm your sense of connection to the Spirit of Life.

# CHAPTER 5

*Is Spiritual Distress Real? Does It*

*Impact Nutrition-Centered Care?*

Being able to decipher the telltale signs of distress of a spiritual nature versus a psychological problem, along with identifying signs of carried or prolonged grief, is helpful for a dietitian or lifestyle medicine provider. This awareness aids the professional in recognizing what type of support would motivate a client and where they may struggle with self-care or follow-through in providing for themselves. Typically, taking care of oneself with healthy food can be more difficult in the throes of malaise, which puts the client more at risk for inadequate nutritional intake, metabolic illness and inflammation.

Interestingly, many clients preferentially seek support and care from dietitians in nutrition counseling and do not arrange to see other providers, like social workers or healthcare chaplains, when they are experiencing spiritual distress.[133] Thus, spiritual and grieving needs may go unaddressed if dietitians do not recognize them and know how to support people experiencing spiritual suffering. Divine struggles and stress impact health and lifestyle behaviors. By providing support in a non-judgmental environment, dietitians can promote healing in the midst of upheaval, which builds trust in nutrition counseling, leads to better follow-through with suggested changes, and ultimately results in better health for the person.

Until now, spirituality has been examined as a positive force in a person's life that aids coping and ideally facilitates finding greater meaning, purpose, identity, and, consequently, well-being or better health. That is the hope, but what happens if a person fails to experience these positive benefits and actually feels the opposite? They may profess belief but at the same time experience a lack of trust in the transcendent in the face of personal or health challenges. Therefore, what if religious or spiritual beliefs become the source of distress and make it more difficult to deal with the health challenge?[134]

Esperandio et al. (2022)[135] expand spiritual distress by classifying it as potentially coming from three areas of life: from interpersonal struggles—struggles between individuals and authority figures, like family members, religious figures, teachers, or coaches who have hurt the person in the past; from intrapersonal struggles—discomfort inside the person, nagging depression, fear, anxiety, scruples, anger, or resentments; and from struggles with divine or transcendent figure thoughts—if there is a loving God, why did my son get sick? Illness and injury tend to isolate people from those who care about them, and they often need help from professionals to reattach or reconnect. Sickness, disability, wounds, chronic conditions, trauma, and major losses all set us apart, at least temporarily.[136]

Knowledge about what constitutes a spiritual struggle can help the practitioner be more aware and sensitive to the patient's needs and even their own difficulties. Typically, being able to invite the client to deeper sharing can help the hidden come to light and relieve troubled energies. The provider in this role functions similarly to a hospital chaplain, not offering therapy but just allowing space and support in light of the difficulty. For some, this might also necessitate a referral to a hospital chaplain or therapist if the experience is complicated or longstanding.

Divine struggles become apparent when the person reports negative feelings, such as anger toward God, disappointment, doubt, or fear focused on God. They may also feel a lack of inner peace, a lack of connectedness to loved ones, an inability to accept what is happening, or an inability to find meaning in life and hope for the future.[137] These individuals may appear sad, desperate, scared, anxious, or angry and may voice loneliness, emptiness, uselessness, guilt, and helplessness, according to Bhatnagar (2017).[138]

The parents of the infant that I described earlier had different reactions to each other. The mother alternated between deep emotional anguish, where she yelled at God for allowing this and seeming numbness, while the father sat frozen the whole time. I just helped by being present with him and did not try to make him emote. Each was experiencing spiritual desolation and deep grief in their own way.

Understanding spiritual distress and the power of supportive presence is important for healthcare practitioners, as there is growing evidence of the harmful effects spiritual distress can have on a person's health and wellness. According to Pagament, Koenig, Tarakeshwar, & Hahn (2001), divine struggle can be "a predictor of increased mortality, even after controlling for demographics, physical health, and mental health factors."[139] Some initial findings show that "greater levels of religious struggles were associated with higher cortisol levels throughout the day" from the insights of Isehunwa (2021),[140] which, in the absence of support, impacts susceptibility to chronic disease and stress-induced illnesses, "depression and poorer quality of life."[141] Research is consistent, too, that when patients experience spiritual distress, along with poor health, they often experience greater physical pain, which is mediated through the "psychoneuroimmunological pathway (interaction between psychological processes and the nervous and immune systems)."[142] Likewise, spiritually-induced stress and depression are "associated with poor appetite, malnutrition, negative gut health, increased cardiovascular disease risk factors, and can lead to a deterioration in glycemic control," according to Riazi et al. (2004).[143]

Spiritual distress and emotional distress often go together, as someone already experiencing emotional upheavals can more easily move to spiritual distress, like the young mother above. Also, certain personality traits may be more often associated with experiencing spiritual distress when problems arise, predisposing people to religious and spiritual distress, such as neuroticism, from the work of Ano & Pargament (2013),[144] trait anger, from Wood et al. (2010),[145] low levels of self-esteem and self-compassion, according to Grubbs, Exline Wilt & Pargament (2014),[146] and a sense of entitlement from Grubbs, Exline & Campbell (2013).[147] This makes discerning the spiritual struggle, as the primary source of the problem, more difficult if the practitioner has not learned to recognize the distinctiveness of spiritual needs and developed a certain spiritual sensitivity in their own experience and life.

In Van Leeuwen's study (2006),[148] often older, more experienced nurses were better able to communicate about a client's divine struggles and spiritual needs. He described that "nurses learn or gain spiritual skills as they interact with patients" and stay in touch with their own reactions. Practitioners of any age can learn these skills if they learn to be alert to life and their own responses in living, which helps them be more compassionate caregivers.

Often, practitioners need to be alert to the sex differences between men and women experiencing divine struggles or distress. Bhatnagar (2017)[149] identified that females were more prone to be spiritually distressed than males, partly because they were slower to assign personal blame to themselves for the illness and were more likely to be angry at God. Men, on the other hand, tended to blame themselves for the difficulty, ascribing bad karma from their own actions as the reason for getting sick. These study participants, interestingly, showed similar assessments of the positive statements about spirituality but differed when in distress. This shows the power of cultural roles and identity.

Particularly interesting to dietitians, nutritionists, and other healthcare team members is the impact of spiritual distress on body image struggles and "compensatory eating behaviors" found by Exline, Homolka, and Harriott (2015).[150] According to Exline et al., compensatory behaviors around eating were purging, fasting, and excessive exercise. These reactive or compensatory behaviors are often understood as "a form of atonement for perceived offenses against God." Body image and eating disorders may stem from an over-emphasis on self-control motivated by a spiritual or religious faith and "may imply a threat of divine punishment for disapproval if standards for good behavior are not met."[151] With this fear in mind, the thinking that if God is displeased with me, how can I like myself predisposes a person to engage in compensatory behaviors in order to shape up.[152] Binging, on the other hand, may be a way to protest a perceived heavy-handed God, a way to escape the wrath after you couldn't meet God's rigid standards.[153]

There were two unexpected findings in Exline's 2015 study. The first was the impact of spiritual distress, even among a sizable portion of non-believers. "25% experienced anger/disappointment towards God, while 16% endorsed some concern about God's disapproval" or negative reactions towards their ideas about God. These results may not be surprising if spirituality is "a biological need helpful for survival," as discussed earlier. What is suggested is that it may be part of human makeup to want somewhere to turn when life is out of control. The other surprise showed that egocentrism and a sense of "having a special relationship with God and a tendency to be manipulative were robust predictors for compensatory behaviors."[154]

What follows is another verbatim account. Notice the themes that surface in the interaction. Do you hear her grieving? Do you notice any spiritual suffering or distress? Would you have approached this the same way? What feelings do you notice inside you as you listen to this conversation?

# An example of addressing spiritual distress:
## The Verbatim Report 2

### I. INFORMATION about the Client:

The patient was a middle-aged woman who came for nutrition support/counseling to gain weight after completing a two-year treatment regime for throat cancer. She had lost 60 lbs. in the last year and was in the 75% of lowest ideal body weight. She has dysphagia and a very sore throat. Her husband had driven her 40 miles to meet with me in person and waited patiently in the car as we met in the clinic. He had been attempting to cook for her but she did not experience much appetite. Prior to the cancer diagnosis, she had worked in the same department for 40 years. She was missing a sense of purpose and the social support of her co-workers who had been bringing food over to her but she was not interacting with them on a daily basis as before. Our visit was a 45-minute follow-up in the family practice clinic.

### II. OBSERVATIONS

What are your feelings going into the encounter? I felt compassion toward the woman. She had been trying to follow through with my recommendations. Her husband appeared generous and was attempting to cook or take her to her favorite restaurants to encourage her intake.

What do you observe about the setting, the person, or the loved ones? She seemed frantic coming, as they had been running late for the session. I experienced a desire to provide a sense of calm for her.

### III. VERBATIM P = Provider CL = Client

Record the visit as you recall it. Include any important non-verbal cues in parenthesis, your inner impressions and your inner dialogue and feelings.

*Example: Try to remember as clear as you can the actual dialogue between you and the client that you want to process. Also note your own feelings and reactions while you worked with the client. Be as honest as you can so you can learn about yourself as you provide care.*

P1: Welcome, good to see you. *I spoke with an intentional soft tone and offered a smile.*

CL1: It's good to be here finally. We got started late and rushed here. I was so afraid we'd be late. My husband's going to wait for us to meet while he stays in the car.

P2. You're here just at the right time. If he'd like to come in and join us, he would be welcome. *It was winter and cold outside.*

CL2: Well, I'm fine. I consider this my time with you and I'll share the information with him. It gives me a break as he seems to be hovering over me all the time. *I wondered if her husband was experiencing some anticipatory grief with her possible life-threatening diagnosis.*

P3: Where would you like to start? *I felt open to her and ready to hear what she had experienced. I could see her emaciated state and the obvious difficulty/pain she was experiencing swallowing. I wanted to weigh her to see if she has stabilized.*

CL3: I get so discouraged with trying to eat. My husband takes me out to my favorite restaurant and encourages me to order what I used to and I can only eat about 1/3 of a cup and it takes me so long to do that. He's so patient with me but I feel like I'm letting him down. He's trying so hard. *I felt worried about her as it would be difficult to stabilize weight with poor intake.*

P3: Well, should we get your weight so you can have some information? She agreed. I weighed her and her weight had not changed from two weeks ago.

CL4: Well, I guess it's better than having my weight go down. I have liked your recipes for those high-calorie snacks and shakes. I have also been supporting my throat with ice cream servings about twice a day. It feels so good on my throat and I feel hungry for it. *I felt relieved that her weight has stabilized and that she had found some helpful snacks.*

P4: That is good news. I'm proud of you. You are working to take care of your body and things have tasted different than they used to. You seem to see that eating right now is something important to do.

CL5: Yes, it's kind of like medicine right now. I feel such pressure when we go out to eat. My husband is sitting across from me watching me eat each mouthful. It takes me so long and I feel kind of self-conscious wearing this scarf on my head since I lost my hair. I look into my husband's eyes and my heart breaks. He loves me so much. *I felt deep sadness envisioning the scene. I felt a tear well up in my eye. As I started to speak next, my voice cracked.*

P5: So you feel close to your husband and his love for you as you sit across from him? Anything else? *I paused in quiet until she spoke.*

CL6: I feel his love and I feel fearful that I'm dying and will not have that time with him. When I can't eat like I used to, I feel panicked and my throat closes up. *She sniffled and wiped a tear from her eyes and sat quietly before me.*

P6: You're feeling really sad with the thought of possibly this signaling the end for you?

CL7: Yes! *She paused a moment.* I just feel like I can tell you anything. Everyone else, the doctors and nurses come in and tell me the facts and never listen to me like you do. I really cherish the time with you! *I felt a deep connection and care for her.*

P7: I'm really glad. I want to provide you with support and what you need. What would help you take care of yourself this next week? We can celebrate that your weight has been stable and that you've had good success eating the high-protein/calorie recipes. Maybe going out with your husband serves another purpose than just calories in? Do you think?

CL8: Yes, I think you are right. Time with my husband is just that, time with him. Regardless of how much I eat right then, I usually take it home and eat several smaller meals out of it. I can add some extra butter to it at home to get more calories too. I was wondering if you had any helpful recipes and websites with high-calorie recipes. I also need to cultivate some renewing actions to turn to when I get anxious. Do you have any ideas on that too?

P8: Should we start with some new recipes and then talk about some renewing activities to support you emotionally?

CL9: Yes. Sounds good. I feel a lot of peace when I work with my hands and when I'm outside. I'm not a churchy person. But the more serious my cancer, I've been thinking that I hope that there is a God and that I've pleased him. *I provided her with some recipes and websites and then thought she would also benefit from speaking with a healthcare chaplain.*

P9: When you work with your hands, you settle down? Are you a crocheter, a knitter an artist? Do you like to color in adult coloring books?

CL10: I learned to crochet when I was a kid but would like to try it again. I also like to work with beads.

P10: *I shared with her the String of Bead project and had her reflect and mention one hope, need or something she was grateful for as she touched a bead.* Maybe after you eat or just before you eat you could get the beads out to ground yourself so your body can better rest and digest?

CL11: That sounds amazing. I will try that and the new recipes. I feel like I have so much on my mind. When can I see you next? *I felt glad that she was experiencing my support and thought additional support would assist her daily coping as well.*

P11: I've enjoyed our time together too and feel glad it was helpful. What would you think about checking on the support group at the oncology clinic that's led by the chaplain? It's not churchy but a place to speak more about what we started talking about today.

CL12: That sounds really helpful. I always thought you had to be a holy roller to go to that group. It's good to know it's for everybody.

## V. EVALUATION & SUPERVISION

Why did you choose this nutrition counseling encounter? I saw how giving her space for feelings opened up a greater capacity to ask deeper questions and allow her to follow through with eating suggestions. By taking the pressure off of herself to eat, she could appreciate her feelings and her husband's feelings toward her.

What are you learning as you record this encounter? Many times, people have not discussed spiritual or renewing activities for self-nurture. I saw how nourishing with food was an offshoot of a greater self-nurturing mindset.

What do you learn about human nature, spirituality, and the Sacred in this encounter? Individuals can experience the impact of the transcendent through ordinary activities that re-center them, i.e., crocheting or knitting.

What social or cultural forces are at work? She was experiencing isolation from the work climate/culture that had nurtured her sense of competence for 40 years.

Where do you want supervision? Was my timing appropriate for referring her to the oncology support group?

What follows is another spiritual assessment tool for you to review and see the impact of illness and spiritual distress. It is intended for a person who is experiencing illness, but you could also review this assessment for yourself. Consider a difficulty of another sort that you may be experiencing, even if it is not illness. Spiritual assessment tools help you develop an inner frame of reference or an ear to listen and to recognize a spiritual need. As you fill out each assessment, notice which one seems to encapsulate the issues most thoroughly.

## SNAP Spiritual Needs Assessment for Patients (Sharma 2012).[155]

### Rate yourself
**5**= Strongly agree, **4**= Agree, **3**= Neither agree nor disagree,
**2**= Disagree, **1**= Strongly Disagree

1.  I have a need to get in touch with other patients with similar illness.

2.  I have a need for relaxation or stress management.

3.  I have a need for learning to cope with feelings of sadness.

4.  I have a need to share my thoughts and feelings with people close.

5.  I have worries about my family.

6.  I have a need to find meaning in my experience of illness.

7.  I have a need to find hope.

8.  I have a need to overcome fears.

9.  I have need for personal meditation or prayer practices.

10. I have a need for relationship with God or something beyond myself.

11. I have a need to become closer to a community of faith.

12. I have a need to cope with any suffering that I'm having.

13. I have a need to find meaning and purpose in living.

14. I have a need to explore death and dying.

15. I have a need to find peace of mind.

16. I have a need to resolve old disputes, hurts or resentments with friends.

17. I have a need to find forgiveness.

18. I have a need to make decisions about my medical treatment consistent with my beliefs/religion.

19. I have a need for a clergy visit from my tradition.

20. I have a need for a visit from a hospital chaplain.

21. I have a need for visits from fellow members of my faith community.

22. I have a need for religious rituals such as chant, prayer, lighting candles or anointing.

23. I have a need for someone to bring me spiritual texts such as the Bible, Quran, Analects of Confucius, Tibetan Book of the Dead.


Total your score. A lower score means lower spiritual need.

# CHAPTER 6

*Is there More for a Dietitian To*

*Understand about Grief? Does Grief*

*Impact Physical Health?*

In many ways, grief parallels what has already been discussed regarding spiritual distress and aligns with the biopsychosocial spiritual dimensions of human experience and health. The reality is that grief impacts all four dimensions of a human being. "The emotions of grief are often experienced as body-felt energies," as noted by Wolfelt & Duvall (2000),[156] as the pain comes from losing the connection to and/or the physical presence of someone or something that sustained and loved us.

Grief is a normal response to the loss of someone or something that we've lost, loved, or valued, which impacts health and personal decision-making. According to Mughal (2024),[157] the "grief experience is not a state, not a disease, but a process" where the griever is "torn apart by the loss" and needs time and assistance to put their life back together. Grieving is "a spiritual journey of the heart and soul."[158] It implies that the person has thoughts and feelings about the person, experience, or thing that they've lost that must come out and reach the surface. This is part of loving someone or something. Each person does this uniquely. Wolfelt parallels this to having a grief box or container that holds these personal responses. Mourning, on the other hand, means that you open the box and bring these feelings, memories, and thoughts to the outside, as "Mourning is grief gone public."[159] This helps the griever "adapt to life after loss," according to Mughal (2024), where difficult feelings do not fester. For the dietitian, this analogy may parallel digestion, as the stomach is a place for holding and digesting. But what happens if the contents do not move through the tract, as in constipation? These torn feelings can get stuck or jammed and cause problems.

The actual issue in the West with grieving, however, is that many people find it very hard to open up and express their personal responses. Wolfelt (2007) suggests that this may be true because we live in "a constant state of urgency," so we do not take the time to be mindful, slow down, and be present. Many dislike the pain of living in "liminal space" or the uncertain period of trying to put life back together. Many want the grieving process to be efficient and relatively painless, which leads to medicating grief feelings away.

Wolfelt (2007) acknowledges the significant role medications play in managing "severe, chronic, disabling conditions." However, there is a tendency to equate the absence of pain and suffering with good mental health. Many individuals learn from their families to fear grief, to minimize and avoid it, or at least to avoid admitting that they cannot cope on their own. If grief is avoided for a long time, it can pose a risk to the body and affect the long-term ability to function, even for those in healthcare professions.

Some people struggle to grieve and mourn because they follow misguided beliefs, thinking that depression, sadness, fear, and pain signify a lack of faith, a failure to please God, or that God has a greater purpose for them than to be with us. This kind of thinking can lead to spiritual distress, as individuals may question why a loving God would allow such suffering. In the medical model, some set time limits for what is considered normal grieving, suggesting that resolution should occur within 6 to 12 months after a loss. Prolonged grief disorder is viewed as continuing acute grief beyond 12 months after death.[160] According to Lundorff (2020), men experience higher levels of acute distress that diminish over time, while women tend to have increasing symptoms of distress over time.[161]

## Terms involved with grief

Specific terms for grief include bereavement, which is the period of grief and mourning following a loss. Anticipatory grief, which affects both the diagnosed individual and their family, occurs in response to an expected loss.[162] Additionally, disenfranchised grief, as noted by Doka (2009), is the grief experienced when a loss is not openly acknowledged, publicly mourned, or socially supported."[163] An example of disenfranchised grief is body grief, a term used primarily by practitioners who work with individuals experiencing disordered eating. This term refers to the feelings of grief a person may feel when their body changes, particularly after weight gain, as discussed in the work of Haupt (2023).[164] This term became more commonly used after the lockdown due to Covid-19. Haupt reports that "50% of Americans gained weight during the pandemic."

Even Elizabeth Kubler-Ross, who pioneered work on grief and wrote *On Death and Dying*, later lamented how grief was commonly described as a linear and sequential process with clearly defined stages (personal conversation, Alan Wolfelt, 2019). According to Wolfelt (2007), working through grief involves "going into the wilderness of grief," where individuals fluctuate between experiences of numbness, anger, bargaining, and denial until they learn to have a new relationship with the deceased that supports them in the present. This process is difficult to define with clear stop points, but the symptoms of prolonged grieving can impede self-care and significantly affect health.

How can the clinician decipher grief from depression or another mental health issue, as some symptoms of grief seem parallel to these other conditions? A more obvious difference is that grieving persons present with yearning and longing for the deceased and preoccupation with thoughts or memories of the deceased (Mughal, 2024), while depression or other mental health issues do not typically show this focus, although there may be times when a person also experiences deep feelings.

## Physical signs of grief

In addition to the intense sadness that can turn into feelings of depression, another telltale sign of grief, according to Wolfelt and Duvall (2009), is "the lethargy of grief" or anhedonia. This describes the sensation a person feels when they lack the strength to attend to their basic needs. The body is wise and will attempt to slow down a person, encouraging them to take time to acknowledge their loss and the feeling of lost control over life. It's important to note that during active grieving, this may not be the right time to provide extensive nutrition and lifestyle education, such as Diabetic Self-Management Education (DSME), as they may lack the focus or retention to engage with it. Keep messages brief.

Grief can manifest as gastrointestinal symptoms. However, these physical symptoms do not always signify medical problems such as dysbiosis, SIBO, or other conditions; rather, they are a part of the grieving process following a significant loss. A person may experience various symptoms, including an empty, acidic stomach, tightness in the throat or chest, digestive issues, noise sensitivity, heart palpitations, nausea, headaches, increased allergy symptoms, changes in appetite, and fluctuations in weight, along with feelings of agitation or overall tension.[165] During active grieving or prolonged grief, it may not be the right time to address gastrointestinal issues through food sensitivity testing, SIBO, or gut microbiome assessments, as grief can cause these symptoms. The only exception is when someone shows signs of a cardiac emergency; while Takotsubo cardiomyopathy (broken heart syndrome) is rare and linked to grief, it necessitates immediate evaluation.

# The movements of grief

When practitioners support people who are grieving, they may observe a range of emotions, transitioning from recognizing their loss to feeling numb, particularly in the early stages. Grievers might experience protest emotions, such as anger that shifts to deep emptiness, sadness, guilt, or remorse.[166] I recall an adult son of a patient who had just learned about his father's death. After I gently shared this news with him, he went outside and punched the hospital wall. Security calmly escorted him to a space where he could regain his composure. This was his first encounter with the new reality of his father's death.

Consider a person who has just been diagnosed with type 2 diabetes and comes to your office feeling very angry. They may not be abusive; rather, they are grieving or protesting a change they never wanted to make. I recall a man in the diabetes center who came to me. He yelled at me and bristled up until I helped him name what he was feeling. The clinician's best approach is to be present and acknowledge their client's feelings, whatever those feelings may be (Wolfelt, 2007), and allow them to experience their emotions.

Grief can create a sense of confusion as individuals struggle to adjust to their new reality. They may feel disorganized, confused, yearning, or even think they see their lost loved one in a crowd. Clients often find nutrition information overwhelming at this point, so suggesting simple strategies to structure their habits and writing them down to post on the refrigerator can be beneficial.

In addition to confusion, many people experience forgetfulness while mourning. If someone forgets why they entered a room or what you just said, it does not necessarily mean they are developing dementia. We can reassure them about this, as many worry about the quality of their memories during periods of bereavement, based on my clinical experience supporting those who are grieving. After a major loss, many people feel an increased sense of anxiety, panic, and fear as these feelings accompany thoughts like, "Will my life have any purpose without this person? I don't think I can live without them."[167] Along with this, sometimes the person swings into feelings of regret and guilt that they could have done something, even though on some level they know this may be false, along with deep feelings of sadness. This dance between sadness, anger, guilt, and numbness indicates that what is happening is normal "soul work," which gradually brings some periods of relief as a movement toward reconciliation. The "relief that comes from acknowledging the pain of grief becomes a critical step toward reconciliation." The person people claim is doing well, holding up without a tear, is the one to be concerned about. The best stance of the clinician, once again, is a non-judgmental, reassuring presence that shows empathy and a non-rushing approach. One dietitian told me about visiting a woman with some nutritional needs in the hospital who had just lost her mother. She supported her by listening and being present with her. She said, "We hardly talked about nutrition, but she hugged me in the end, saying she got so much out of it, and now she had an appetite." Spiritual care within the nutrition practice often requires more listening than having all the wisdom or information to share.

Reconciliation of the loss does not mean they won't have grief bursts or feel sad when something touches them as a reminder of their loss, and they have intense, albeit short, snaps of feelings. Integration of the pain comes when "the pain of grief goes from being ever-present, sharp, and stinging to an acknowledged feeling of loss that has given rise to renewed meaning and purpose."[168] The reconciliation of grief hopefully brings one back to a positive spirituality, at their own speed, sooner rather than later. As Alan Wolfelt & Duvall (2009) say, "They have to go back before they can go forward" and "there are no rewards for speed."

As you listen to the grieving person, ask yourself: What is the person teaching me about where they are in the process of coming to terms with the loss? Do I need to respect their numbness and allow them some time, or are they self-medicating with something, even comfort food, that I could help them recognize and bring forward? How can I help them create a safe place here so they can open or peek into the grief box? Being numb, angry, or disbelieving can be a sign of healthy grieving.

Mourning has to be dosed, meaning that it's best not to force them to confront the loss until they give you signs that this is what they need. I remember the justified anger towards me early in my training from a family member in the emergency room after I invited him to express his feelings about his mother's death after just learning about it. My responses were attempts to *do this right* but I was not respecting his need to feel numbness for a time. The goal is to learn how to accompany someone with their loss and responses, not to solve their problems. Clinicians need to open their own "emotional and grief box" and make sure they don't have unaddressed needs that will make walking alongside someone else in pain difficult.

Practitioners can be invaluable not by having many words but by just sitting with the person who is distraught and, when they are ready, inviting them to share something about the person they are grieving. Ask them, "What was he like? Where did you meet, and what did you like about him?" These questions invite the person to remember, feel, and share in the safety of a caring relationship. When they are ready, from my clinical experience, most people appreciate being able to say the person's name and share their story.

## Physical changes in grieving

In the throes of active grief, the body is vulnerable to certain maladies, as all systems of the body are affected, particularly the immune and cardiovascular systems. For example, in an older study by Young (1963), 4,486 widowers who were compared to married men were found to have "a 40% increase in mortality rate in the first 6 months of bereavement with little differential thereafter."[169] From the work of Edmondson (2013),[170] it is noted that during intense grief, many show an increase in proinflammatory cytokines, as well as other hemodynamic changes, including increased blood pressure, increased heart rate, arrhythmias, increased platelet activity and aggregation, increased release of endothelin (a protein that increases vasoconstriction), and increased production of fibrinogen, which promotes plaque destabilization and the prothrombotic state. Intense emotions were also tied to increases in catecholamine release and increased sympathetic nervous system activation according to Mughal.[171] These effects lessened somewhat over time for those effectively grieving but remained impactful for those experiencing prolonged grief reactions. Grievers are prone to higher blood pressure and a greater likelihood of heart attacks and strokes, depending on their individual predispositions and levels of inflammation.

Many studies concur that in early stages of loss, and with stress, levels of cortisol were chronically increased, for at least the first 6 months, by as much as 30% as compared to the nonbereaved[172] and "the cortisol: DHEA ratio was elevated, especially for men."[173] According to Buckley, DHEA is an immune enhancer and as adults age, less is released from the hypothalamic-pituitary-adrenal axis. Therefore, the immune systems of older men are especially negatively impacted by "chronically elevated levels of cortisol, showing increased cardiac risk, reduced immune function and reduced quality of life." [174] [175]

Grief specifically impacts the production and effectiveness of immune cells, particularly during active grieving. A study of individuals actively grieving found lower numbers of T-cells and natural killer cells at 2 weeks, 6 weeks, 1 month, and 12 months post-loss, as seen in the work of Kanfer[176] and Schleifer.[177] In contrast, the number of neutrophils (nonspecific inflammatory cells) increased, but their ability to function in raising an inflammatory response to pathogens decreased. This reduced immune function was prolonged and significantly noted in individuals exhibiting symptoms of complicated or dysfunctional grief, specifically those showing "harm-avoidant personality traits and a long-lasting dysphoric mood following the unexpected death of their spouse," according to Gerra,[178] as cited in Buckley.[179] They also showed greater suppression of immune responses to pathogens than their normally grieving counterparts, suggesting that coping styles may impact immune function.

Grieving individuals are more prone to strokes and heart attacks due to thrombosis and worsening existing cardiac problems, as well as conditions negatively affected by inflammation and stress. They also have a reduced capacity to fight infections. Young people may find it easier to navigate short-term changes, but older individuals face increased risks for known cardiovascular diseases. Takotsubo cardiomyopathy, also known as broken heart syndrome, is a real condition. This cardiomyopathy, characterized by a weakening of the left ventricle leading to ballooning, is 90% more likely to occur in women, especially in post-menopausal women, in the advent of intense loss.[180]

Interestingly, being present and participating in support groups can lower cortisol levels, decrease doctor visits, and stabilize CD4 cell counts, according to Goodkin (1998), as cited in Buckley (2012),[181] especially for patients with compromised immune systems prior to the loss, such as patients with HIV.

Each member of the healthcare team is responsible for promoting the health of individuals who are actively grieving and those who are dealing with unprocessed grief.

According to Mughal (2024), providers must develop empathetic communication and remain attentive to specific aspects of patient care within their disciplines. For dietitians, it is essential to guide clients toward anti-inflammatory foods and dietary practices that support heart health, monitor salt intake, and address nutrient needs that influence blood pressure and glucose management. Additionally, dietitians should encourage adherence to daily self-care routines focused on healthy whole foods, sleep hygiene, and stress management, while being mindful of the client's connections to their support networks for emotional and spiritual uplift.

## Important ramifications for nutritional health during grieving

Johnson (2002) shows the importance of addressing issues with food following a recent bereavement, as bereaved persons showed common struggles in taking care of themselves through eating healthy food, and have a significant risk of nutritional deficits following a recent loss. For couples, the risk of poor nutrition was lower but still present. Bereavement counseling did not reduce this risk for the 22 individuals who completed a questionnaire assessing dietary intake, eating behavior, and food handling. The majority, regardless of whether they received bereavement counseling, exhibited poor eating behaviors that placed them at moderate risk for poor nutrition, scoring above 3.[182] The coupled group had the lowest risk of nutritional deficiency. These common dietary issues included problems with:

1. Food acquisition, preparation and consumption

2. Difficult meal place and time

3. Difficult influence of social network/spouse

4. Food and nutrition information.[183]

Although emotional counseling/therapy did not reduce the risk of poor nutritional intake, considering their struggles with isolation and a weak social network, a possible source of support could be small group sessions with peers or the supportive presence that spiritual care from the practitioner provides.

Additionally, grieving individuals face challenges with purchasing and cooking healthy foods, understanding nutrition information, and often dislike eating alone. They may also be particularly physically vulnerable to the negative effects of highly processed, nutrient-deficient foods due to the physical adaptations associated with the grieving process. Research indicates that grieving interacts with dietary behaviors.[184] Psychological stress and low moods increase cravings for high-fat comfort foods and fast food. In a study involving 58 widowed older adults, researchers found that those who were grieving consumed twice as many commercial meals weekly compared to their non-grieving peers. This included fast food, high-carbohydrate/sugar comfort foods, and prepackaged processed meals, resulting in a nutritional deficit score that was more than twice as high as that of married, non-grieving adults.[185] They also demonstrate an enhanced triglyceride response to a high-saturated fat meal, with a 14% slower clearance of triglycerides from the blood.[186] Grievers seem more vulnerable to infections and illnesses due to changes in the immune system caused by grief. Therefore, recommending good hygiene practices, such as handwashing, can be particularly helpful.

## Signs of carried grief and catch-up mourning

If the pain of loss goes unhealed, it drains enthusiasm for living and stifles creativity, meaning, and purpose. Look for signs of pronounced symptoms, which Wolfelt (2009) calls "fallout symptoms of carried grief." Make a mental note to listen for these and include them in your initial and ongoing assessments. Symptoms that persist over time and do not seem to lessen include difficulties with trust and intimacy, depression and a negative outlook, anxiety and panic attacks, psychic numbing and disconnection, irritability and agitation, substance abuse, addictions, eating disorders, and physical problems, whether real or imagined.[187] Some say these symptoms describe the "loss of the divine spark." Do they seem to enshrine the person they're grieving, dwell excessively on them, and hold onto reminders of them? Remember the signs of positive spirituality and notice if they are consistently missing.

I remember one patient in inpatient addiction recovery who wore a necklace containing her husband's ashes for the last five years and brought his photos to our sessions. Another dietitian told me about a patient who was grieving her daughter and became fixated on losing weight, even though she did not carry extra weight and had not previously struggled with eating issues before her daughter's death. The dietitian remarked, "It was as if, by losing weight and controlling her body, she felt a sense of control over something." This illustrates how she focused on physical aspects when her true need was to express her deep feelings. Wolfelt recommends assisting a client with "catch-up mourning," the process of revisiting and grieving losses that may not have been fully processed. He states, "When we learn to be with the pain that we have denied, we retrieve those parts of ourselves that were left behind." It is as if, to have "a psychologically rich life," as described earlier, we must go back, open the box, and engage in this mourning.

Wolfelt suggests using a four-part model for addressing carried grief, which dietitians can keep in mind when their patients show signs of it. First, the person must acknowledge their grief, often sharing it with a trusted individual. Dietitians (RDs) can play this role, as patients frequently share intimate details like their bowel habits—so why not this as well?

Second, they need to overcome their resistance to talking about the loss. RDs can encourage them to share what they're feeling, exercising patience and understanding that processing past losses is a sign of trust and the only way forward. Some individuals, particularly quiet introverts, may mourn internally without overt displays of emotion.

Third, they actively confront the grief they have been carrying. For instance, a 35-year-old might cry when speaking about his grandfather who died when he was 10. This is a healing process!

Finally, fourth, they begin to integrate their grief, as discussed earlier. Their emotions settle down, becoming episodes in an otherwise positive life. When someone is actively grieving or stuck in the "ghosts of grief" from the past, dietitians can best serve this population by listening more than speaking and keeping nutritional information simple, practical, and based on the clients' ability to process new information.

As providers focused on lifestyle and nutrition and its positive effects on health, dietitians and lifestyle medicine providers should remember that "it is only when we care for ourselves physically that we can integrate our losses emotionally and spiritually," according to Wolfelt.[188] Dietitians often hear about challenges faster than other providers because they spend more time assessing patients' coping strategies, emotional and physical symptoms, and the quality of their daily self-care routines. Within a healthcare or interdisciplinary team, sharing insights about a patient's self-care behaviors, moods, and perceptions can greatly improve care. The dietitian's role is to teach the skills of personal guardianship or responsibility that individuals need to manage their unique needs during the grieving process. A perceptive nutrition or lifestyle medicine professional may model and promote this holistic approach among practitioners from different disciplines.

What follows is a personal reflection activity and the Carried Grief Scale by Dr. Allan Wolfelt. Before a practitioner can adequately attend to the deep feelings and experiences of loss in another's life, they must be aware of their own needs and unfinished or carried grief in their own lives. Complete both now prior to Part 2 of this resource, where the clinical process formation/education activities will be described.

**Personal Reflection**

Read "A Healthy Path to Long-Term Healing" by Dr. Allan Wolfelt to reflect on your own response to grief. Access the article at centerforloss.com.

Think about someone or something you have lost. It may have been years ago, but you might still be carrying that loss.

Gently let thoughts and memories about that person, experience, or relationship come to the surface. What do you miss, value, or long for? What does this reveal about yourself, your life, and your values?

Express these feelings and memories: draw a picture, write a poem, or look at an old photo and appreciate the scene. Find a friend or a journal page to share the feelings that arise.

Be gentle and let this experience unfold.

## The Carried Grief Self-Inventory[189]

This assessment is designed to help the person (the practitioner) consider the sources of carried pain that they experience. "The purpose of this inventory is not to shame or discourage you but to empower you."

Use the following list to remind yourself of people or things, or capacities that you grieve or lost, where you might still carry some pain. Look over the list and check or circle the ones that apply to you in your own life. The list is not comprehensive, so feel free to write in others at the end of the inventory. First, you will inventory what type of losses you have experienced and second assess any symptoms of carried grief that you notice in yourself.

## Loss of People You Love

Separation (physical and or emotional)

Rejection

Hostility/grudges

Illness (Alzheimer's, debilitating condition)

Divorce

Abandonment/betrayal

Death

Empty nest

## Loss of Pets

## Loss of Aspects of Self

Self-esteem (sometimes through physical, or sexual or emotional abuse, rape, humiliation, rejection or neglect)

Health (physical or mental, or mental ability)

Job (downsizing, firing, failed business, retirement)

Control (addiction, victimization, eating disorder)

Innocence (abuse, exposure to immoral behavior)

Sexual identity/ability/desire

Security (financial problems, war)

Expectations (about how life should or would or ought to be)

Reputation

Beliefs (religious, spiritual, belief in trusted others)

Dreams (cherished hopes for the future)

## Loss of Physical Objects

Home (through physical disaster, move or transition into assisted-living environment)

Linking objects (cherished photos, jewelry etc.)

Money

Belongings (theft, fire)

Nature/place (with a move or changing land use)

## Loss through Developmental Transitions

Toddlerhood to childhood

Childhood to adolescence

Adolescence to adulthood

Leaving home

Marriage

Having a child/ not having a child

Mid-life

Care-giving of parents

Retirement

Old age

## Other losses:

## A summary of my major losses:

**After inventorying your loses, go another step by answering the following questions. Circle the response that is honestly most like you.[190] For more resources, go to the Center for Loss and Life Transitions, Fort Collins, CO.**

1.    Do you have difficulties with trust and intimacy?
      Never          Seldom          Occasionally          Often          Usually

2.    Do you have a tendency toward depression and a negative outlook?
      Never          Seldom          Occasionally          Often          Usually

3.    Do you have difficulties with anxiety and/or panic attacks?
      Never          Seldom          Occasionally          Often          Usually

4.    Do you have trouble with psychic numbing and disconnection?
      Never          Seldom          Occasionally          Often          Usually

5.    Do you have difficulties with irritability and agitation?
      Never          Seldom          Occasionally          Often          Usually

6.    Do you struggle with substance abuse?
      Never          Seldom          Occasionally          Often          Usually

7.    Do you have any physical problems, real or imagined?
      Never          Seldom          Occasionally          Often          Usually

8.  Do you see yourself living out aspects of grief avoidance responses?

    Never        Seldom        Occasionally        Often        Usually

9.  Do you find it easier to take care of others than you do to care for yourself?

    Never        Seldom        Occasionally        Often        Usually

10. Do you find it difficult to express your feelings?

    Never        Seldom        Occasionally        Often        Usually

11. Do you find it difficult to ask for what you want from other people?

    Never        Seldom        Occasionally        Often        Usually

12. Do you feel a lack of meaning and purpose in your life?

    Never        Seldom        Occasionally        Often        Usually

If you answered "Occasionally," "Often," or "Usually" to any of these questions, you are probably experiencing symptoms of carried grief. Recognizing, acknowledging, and personally mourning these losses will take some time and be best done with support of trusted friend, counselor, or faith leader.

# CHAPTER 7

*Can a Practitioner Be More Effective with Clients when they Assess Spiritual Needs?*

Research shows that patients prefer to receive support from practitioners they see more frequently.[191] In a study with cancer patients (n=1,213), patients' psychosocial needs were assessed at the second oncology visit. Sixty-three percent of patients who needed a referral saw the dietitian, while 37% of those patients did not meet the criteria to see the RD but saw them anyway.[192] Consistent with prior data from Pearce et al. (2012) and others, a diagnosis of cancer triggered higher utilization of psychological services, specifically referrals to dietitians, in preference to chaplaincy care.[193] In Hamilton's (2018) study, of all patients seeking psychosocial support, 30% saw a dietitian while only 5% sought out the chaplain. Various factors may have contributed to this discrepancy, including a lack of availability of chaplains. However, it is evident that many cancer patients experienced spiritual needs, and if the dietitian did not address these, they were likely left unaddressed.

## Addressing spiritual needs matters to patients

Patients, especially those with serious illnesses, consider religion important; about 88% do, according to Balboni.[194] Ninety-one percent are aware of their spiritual needs, as noted by Pearce[195] while 58% want their physicians and healthcare team to ask them about their spirituality, according to Astrow.[196] Balboni reported disappointing results in this later study which showed that most patients with advanced cancer, however, never received spiritual support from their nurses (86%) or physicians (87%).[197] The strongest predictor for the healthcare team to offer spiritual support was the professional development focused on spiritual care. If most patients consider religion important and want their providers to engage with them about these spiritual needs during a serious illness, why aren't care providers doing this?

Maybe it's lack of time, or that the providers do not think this is in their wheelhouse, but as we have seen, avoiding addressing these needs impacts the patient's health and satisfaction with their care. Startlingly, according to Pearce et al, even after the "91% of patients at a southeastern medical center with advanced cancer desired and received spiritual care from their healthcare providers, 17% of these still desired more. According to these patients, what they received from the healthcare team was not adequate to meet their needs. Seriously ill patients who receive insufficient spiritual support report increased physical pain, higher depression scores, and greater mortality from their illness according to Giese-Davis.[198] Spiritual care appears to matter to patients, but providers seem to be falling short.

## How to begin to address spiritual needs?

By now, the importance of listening to the patient's narrative is clear. Hearing and understanding the person's life and culture is essential for practitioners caring for distressed individuals. Otherwise, they might overlook important spiritual and psychosocial factors affecting the person's reactions and health. It's crucial to encourage the person to discuss how their illness has impacted them, how they once found meaning, and how the illness has influenced their perceptions of God or their spiritual practices. Do they view this illness as unfair or as a consequence of their own poor choices? Asking whether they wish to connect with a spiritual leader can reveal their stance on spirituality. Additionally, be attentive to compensatory behaviors such as purging and bingeing, and gently inquire about their feelings toward God and themselves.

## An initial framework for spiritual screening

Spiritual screens, or short spiritual history inventories, are surface assessments best used to identify serious or emergent spiritual needs in patients. This allows for referrals to a spiritual leader, healthcare chaplain, or timely contact with a faith leader for those who are strongly religious, in my clinical opinion. Many individuals with spiritual concerns who consider themselves religious often respond negatively to these questions because they do not recognize their needs as spiritual. While spiritual screens can help identify significant spiritual issues, patients typically have not yet received supportive presence or spiritual care when these tools are used. They primarily serve as "getting started questions." Dietitians do not need to stop at this point; once trained, they can listen for spiritual issues, offer supportive presence, and follow up with mind/body/spiritual practices that align with the person's culture, which aids in healing.

Nurses, physicians and other healthcare team members may also frequently ask about these initial needs. Instruments like the FICA,[199] the HOPE,[200] or the Mattering Tool[201] ask basic questions like: Are you religious or spiritual, and how important is this to you? What gives you hope? Are you part of a faith community? How would you like this to impact your care here? Using these simple questions, I was able to recognize the need and arrange for a Native American faith leader to come to the nursing home to burn sacred sage for a Native American patient (which set off the fire alarm). I had to do more active listening to encourage the patient to speak about his carried grief that was impacting his appetite after he was removed from his community into the nursing home.

To assess spiritual needs, Lycett (2020) proposes a simple spiritual screening process.[202] The dietitian is encouraged to incorporate the gathered information into their nutrition assessment, identified nutrition problems, planning, and monitoring processes. The purpose of this initial screening is to broadly identify individuals who may be experiencing immediate spiritual or religious distress that requires urgent attention. Dietitians should ask and document responses to the following questions:

1.  Do you consider yourself spiritual or religious?

2.  How do your beliefs or values influence what
    you eat or how you manage/cope with your health?

3.  Do you have any spiritual or religious concerns at this time?

These questions play an important role, as many patients later find an open door to share with dietitians highly emotive issues in their lives beyond just their eating habits or exercise routines. These patients often do not seek support from spiritual leaders. Bottled-up distress, grief, and the need for support and spiritual care can have health impacts, as we have explored. Additionally, dietitians, after considering the insights from a spiritual screening, can start to listen for spiritual needs, distress, and signs of active and lingering grief. The second portion of this resource will continue to help you provide more comprehensive supportive spiritual care that is centered in your discipline.

As a nutrition or lifestyle medicine professional, you can engage patients more deeply to help those who may not recognize their struggles as spiritual to work through obstacles and receive support, enabling them to move forward with lifestyle medicine. You do not need to be a specialist or religious leader to engage patients deeply; you can remain within your discipline. Listen for the compelling aspects of their narratives, noting what is most important to them, which can serve as an asset in promoting healthy self-care. Observe how they recharge, energize themselves, and nourish their spirit and motivation to maintain positive self-care behaviors and habits. Ask yourself, 'How do they flourish, and what motivates them to get out of bed in the morning?' Listen for clues related to the dimensions of spirituality, meaning, purpose, and well-being to identify what is most compelling or helpful for their healing journey. Consider what they wish to share and where they might benefit from your emotional support. Responding to these insights provides a valuable way to integrate spiritual care into your nutritional counseling and healthcare practice.

Spiritual assessment begins with attentive listening to the details. What you seek requires keen listening and deciphering skills. It's often similar to driving down a road. In my area, there's a peculiar practice of camouflaging cell phone towers; they often resemble odd pine trees. In Phoenix, they mimic palm trees, designed as metal poles topped with metallic palm fronds to disguise their true nature. They appear strangely out of place until you recognize what they are. Spiritual assessment can sometimes feel like this, as you notice what is positive and what seems amiss. When you pay attention, you'll catch it.

After this following verbatim, in the next chapter, we will explore how to apply spiritual care principles in complex situations. For example, a current hot topic, VSED or the Voluntary Stopping of Eating and Drinking, is something a person may request help from a dietitian or lifestyle medicine provider to implement when they are experiencing spiritual distress. Codes of Ethics for each healthcare profession are fashioned to guide practitioners to reason out appropriate and morally right professional actions when it is unclear. Dignity therapy, a unique form of spiritual support, will be described as another spiritual care technique for the non-chaplain healthcare providers' tool box.

Consider this next verbatim, which describes how spiritual care can be included inside of nutrition care. Consider if you would have engaged differently with the client and why. What feelings surface inside of you as you reflect on this. Which aspect or definition of spirituality seems to fit this person? What aspects of grief are impacting this person? What are they using to cope with the loss? Are they at nutritional risk? What carries this risk in their lifestyle? Consider any ways you might side-step an issue for the client that you have not dealt with in yourself. With these types of insights, you will be able to examine them in the second portion of this work when we look at the "transformative learning process."

## An example of grief inside of a clinical visit:
## The Verbatim Report 3

I. INFORMATION about the Client: He was completing the last week of the 10-week intensive treatment program for substance abuse and received a new diagnosis of type He was identified by his therapist as having nutritional issues. The visit took place in a chemical dependency outpatient clinic. This was the initial visit.

### II. OBSERVATIONS

What are your plans and anticipations with this person/loved one(s)? I want to offer an open-ended experience to provide support/nutrition education for healthy lifestyle in response to this patient's needs. I am not aware of an agenda other than to listen attentively to him and to respond to his needs.

What are your feelings going into the encounter? I feel relaxed, ready and open.

What do you observe about the setting, the person, or the loved ones? He seems open, comfortable talking with me, as I have been attending large group sessions with the group for the last several weeks. We utilize one of my co-worker's offices as is protocol, as I do not have my own office.

### III. VERBATIM P = Provider, CL = Client

Record the visit as you recall it. Include any important non-verbal cues in parenthesis, your inner impressions and your inner dialogue and feelings.

Example: Try to remember as clear as you can the actual dialogue between you and the client. Also note your own feelings, reactions and your own inner dialogue while you worked with the client. Be as honest as you can so you can learn about yourself as you provide care.

P1: Hi PL, can we take a minute to talk? *I feel open to begin working one-on-one, and I am curious what this interaction will involve.*

CL1: Yes, that would be fine. (We walk from the group room, across the hall to the staff offices.)

P2: I'm an office moocher because I don't have my own office. We'll meet in here. (I chuckle and unlock the door and we sit across from each other.)

CL2: I'm really glad to get a chance to talk with you. I've got many issues the doctor wants me to change in how I'm living. It is difficult as I have a lot on my mind. I've had so much happen to me in the last few years with three family members dying in one year and my favorite dog dying too. I'm really mad at God right now. I don't know how I'm going to change what I eat.

P3: Yes, sounds like so much is on your mind. Where do you want to start? *I felt compassionate toward him.*

CL3: Yes, two years ago, my mom got sick and died from stomach cancer and a heart problem. I was really close to her. She was the warmth in our family. My dad really did care but he never could show it. I don't think that I ever heard him say that he loved me. But my mom did. At my mom's funeral, my brother stumbled at the graveside, which I thought was odd. He always was the healthy one, not like me with all these medical problems growing up. But to top it all off, two months later he died suddenly from a heart attack. *I felt care toward him and thought he wanted support and some simple education. I wanted to show focused attention toward him during our session.*

P4: No warning at all and he was gone too! You were left with a lot to handle, weren't you.

CL4: Yes, I felt immobilized with this sadness. That is when I really started using and I turned my back on God. If you do that kind of thing to me, God, I can't trust you. I guess I'll just do my own thing. That seemed to work but I still had all this stuff happening to me, giving me more sense that God was not protecting me—like the diabetes! *I noticed tears welling up in his eyes. There was silence for a moment.*

P5: You sound like you got angry toward God and frustrated with your situation, like there was nowhere to turn. *I wondered if he has ever grieved all this compounded loss, just used drugs to stuff the feelings.* Do you wonder if us getting a chance to speak is a way God is providing for you now? *I felt open to his feelings and story.*

CL5: Well, maybe, I never looked at it that way. I've got to start taking care of myself!

P6: Should we talk about what you can do to take care of yourself?

CL6: Yes, I want to know where to start to kick this diabetes.

P7: Well, let's start by you telling me what you usually eat for meals. When you were using, tell me about your meals.

Cl 7: (He gave a brief 24 recall of his usual meals.) I want two ideas I can try like cutting out sugar pop and not snacking at night cuz I know those aren't good with diabetes.

P8: So, you will cut out pop and replace it with ___ and cut out nighttime snacking as often as you can, and do what instead at least three times a week?

CL8: (He decided he would play the guitar three times a week instead of snacking.) I will drink sparkling water three times per week instead of soda pop. I bet my mom and brother would be proud of me that I'm doing that.

P9: *I noticed that he circled back to his grief and loss. I realized that untended grief if delved into can sometimes trigger a relapse behavior but since he brought that up, I would use that thought to help reinforce his behavior change.* Yes, and if thoughts of your mom or brother come to your mind, you could welcome them and savor what they meant to you. We can share about that too next week.

## V. EVALUATION & SUPERVISION

Why did you choose this encounter? This was a prime example of spiritual distress right in the middle of nutrition counseling. I saw him willing to speak of his loss and the anger toward God which seemed to open him up to trying some strategies to manage his diabetes. He seemed like he felt heard, nurtured and understood when I listened to his concerns.

What are you learning as you record this encounter? I learned that allowing conversations about God and spiritual distress created openness in him to tackle lifestyle change. I had to keep it simple as I perceived carried grief.

What did you learn about human nature, spirituality and the sacred in this encounter? I recognized the unity between physiological, emotional and spiritual responses.

What social or cultural forces are at work? He valued family connections and had abused substances when his emotional and social needs were not met in intimate human relationships. This lack seemed to alienate him from God.

Where do you want supervision? Did I move to information giving too soon as based on my own history of experiencing the death of my mother?

# CHAPTER 8

*Embracing the Fullness*

*of the Hippocratic Oath:*

*Understanding Ethics in*

*Complex Cases*

Maybe you were like me when I first started considering ethics for Registered Dietitians. You were interested, but the whole topic seemed daunting and less than engaging, leaving you with the question, "Why are ethics important for nutrition and dietetics?" Ethics are guiding principles that help ensure that professionals offer care that safeguards people's health. Dietitians take the Hippocratic oath, which emphasizes several key and distinct components that we will explore here.

There are many reasons to have ethical standards to guide the practice of nutrition and dietetics. We live in complex times, and to provide appropriate care consistent with our value systems, we have to be able to reason complicated situations out and determine the best response. This is the essence of being a responsible professional. Patients rely on and trust us to provide care for their benefit.

If we explore the Hippocratic oath, it is based primarily on two important principles: the principle of beneficence, or the premise that the physician or the dietitian, within the limits of their ability and judgment, is always to act for the patient's good. The second premise is that the practitioner is to do no harm or show non-maleficence. Physicians have followed the Hippocratic oath for 2,500 years, as it was devised in the 4th to 5th century BC.[203]

Over the years, this oath has also evolved to include the necessity for all health professionals to work to prevent disease and promote the health knowledge and skills of each other on the healthcare team and for patients. For dietitians, this means that we use the evidence from the literature to assess and address health through our expertise in nutrition and lifestyle medicine. We serve the healthcare team by sharing this knowledge and skill set.

Let's explore the current Code of Ethics for the Nutrition and Dietetics Profession from 2018. We see that these standards support the Hippocratic oath and are articulated in four principles of practice. They state that nutrition and dietetic professionals are to practice "non-maleficence" or are to take "an evidence-based approach" to use "in-depth scientific knowledge of food, human nutrition, and behavior to make evidence-based decisions for the benefit of the patient.

In addition, they are to practice "professionalism" or beneficence, to "participate in and contribute to decisions that affect the well-being of patients or clients."[204] This includes acting justly with other team members, professions, and people the RD supervises, to "contribute to the advancement and competence of others, including colleagues, students, and the public," according to this previously mentioned statement from the Academy in 2018.

Two other dimensions of ethics, acting justly and supporting patient autonomy, are to work in a balanced fashion with the principles of beneficence and non-maleficence. Dietitians must respect patients' autonomy by safeguarding confidentiality and providing and documenting accurate information. Likewise, they are to avoid conflicts of interest and comply with requirements for maintaining their credentials. In addition, nutrition professionals are to promote justice and work to reduce health disparities, provide "fair and equitable treatment" to patients, and offer community service that promotes "the public's trust in the profession."

While understanding these basic principles may seem helpful, a pressing issue arises for the nutrition professional when these four principles become misaligned or unhinged. Problems arise when the principle of patient autonomy becomes primary and over-shadows other aspects of ethical care. This is particularly important for the rather recent issue of VSED, or Voluntarily Stopping Eating and Drinking.

VSED is not the withholding of food and drink for people who are actively dying or for those experiencing adverse consequences from assisted nutrition (tube feeding or TPN) that cannot be rectified. Here, assisted nutrition presents an undue burden to the human system and can ethically be withheld because it presents further suffering and risk to the person in the form of aspiration pneumonia, etc. What's more, according to the Medical-Moral Commission from the Archdiocese of Dubuque (2024), "medically assisted nutrition and hydration becomes morally optional when they cannot reasonably be expected to prolong life or would be excessively burdensome for the patient" by resulting in medical complications.

VSED is when patients seek to hasten their own death when they determine that life is not worth living. This could be in light of a chronic, debilitating illness that, down the road, they do not want to or don't think that they can deal with. In Clinical Guidelines for Voluntarily Stopping Eating and Drinking,[205] VSED is defined as "a deliberate, self-initiated action by a patient with decision-making capacity to hasten death in the setting of suffering refractory to optimal palliative interventions, or suffering due to an irreversible illness, that the person regards as unacceptable."

This means that a competent, capacitated person voluntarily and deliberately stops eating and drinking with the "primary intention of hastening death because of the persistence of unacceptable suffering."[206] These patients often approach healthcare professionals, including dietitians, to facilitate this action.

The question remains in making this decision: do they have full freedom to make life-altering decisions? Is any fear, misinformation, sense of isolation etc., limiting or coloring their choice?

Consider your response to a patient who approaches you with suicide ideation. At this moment, due to depression, discouragement, loneliness, or another stressor they do not think they can cope with, they want to end their life. What are you obligated to do here as a responsible professional? Would it be to help them be safe and articulate what is bothering them or discourage them from taking such a drastic action? In this light, are people with suicide ideation able to exercise their full freedom of choice?

Contrary to this thinking of providing support and keeping people safe when they are in the depths of despair, the clinical guidelines from Wechkin et al. are meant to guide how providers promote and discuss VSED as an option and how they provide care to these patients while they undergo VSED. Ortiz presents clearly the ethical problems of doing so. VSED is legal in all of the USA because it is considered "passive euthanasia." However, the question that remains for dietitians is whether discussing and supporting patients to choose VSED is consistent with a balanced understanding of the Code of Ethics for Nutrition and Dietetic professionals.

Why is this important for the dietitian to understand? Dietitians want to provide ethical patient care and counsel other team members on these issues. Eating and drinking are our primary focus. We must apply these four ethical principles in balance with each other to decipher best practices concerning VSED. Self-autonomy is one aspect of ethical care that must be exercised in balance with doing no harm and keeping the patient's best interests at heart.

First, from an ethical perspective, eating and drinking are considered the ordinary or normal care of a person. It is not a treatment or considered medical care or life-prolonging intervention. Consistent with ethics, giving food and water is in the same realm as providing shelter and clothing. This is the essence of providing just care.

Supporting basic care of the human person is the essence of doing no harm and keeping the patient's best interests in mind.

Many times, when patients are adjusting and coping with significant medical issues, they "may be anxious, depressed or not able to see past the present situation."[207] Although legal, some health decisions are morally wrong, both for the patient and the professional to explain and be involved with in providing patient care. Presenting VSED as an option, explaining it, and being involved in offering palliative care during the self-chosen course of VSED breaks patient-provider trust and undermines the basic tenets of the Hippocratic oath and ethical practice of "do no harm" and keeping the health and well-being of the patient in mind.

In caring for the critically or chronically ill person, providers must not forget that there is a "given degree of psychological dependency of a very ill patient on his doctor (or dietitian) and the potential for subtle and unintentional influence that is troubling."[208] Thus, honoring the patient's decision to take their own life places autonomy over all other ethical parameters and makes the provider complicit in a morally unacceptable act.

Interestingly, there is very little research into why a person chooses VSED. Right now, the law does not mandate that a person requesting to end their life through VSED be evaluated for depression or mental health concerns. Here is a primary area where the dietitian must trigger the entire team to assess and address the patient's needs, just like they would with anyone expressing suicide ideation instead of participating in the patient's death wish. As Otiz expresses, "A human life is at stake, and the patient needs to be listened to, cared about, and affirmed." Many physicians and nurses have limited time due to the length of their typical visits, while dietitians have much longer appointment times with patients.

It is imperative for dietitians to understand some simple practices to offer spiritual or existential care in these situations to address the spiritual or dignity-related distress that motivates a request for VSED. A specific tool like the Patient Dignity Inventory is helpful in guiding the practitioner in discussing the patient's concerns. The PDI is a rather new instrument with 25 questions that get to the heart of what is distressing the person, including spiritual distress, dependency, peace of mind, and social support. Topics covered in this instrument cover a wide range of concerns, including physical, psychosocial, existential, and spiritual facets of the patient experience. Most report that even the most terminally ill patient can complete the inventory in 1–2 minutes.[209] Any nutrition or dietitian professional working with critically ill, palliative care, or any patients struggling with distress needs to become familiar with this simple instrument. This allows them to understand human suffering more fully and how to deliver dignity-conserving care to enable patients to articulate what ordinarily is hard to speak about.

Another simple method devised by Chochinov, if a provider does not have experience with using the simple yet full 25-item Patient Dignity Inventory, is to ask one question: "What do I need to know about you as a person to give you the best care possible?" Evidence shows that even this simple inquiry helps patients feel heard and increases the provider's compassion and understanding of the patient's needs.[210]

It is interesting to note that "the care of the sick unfolds in stories," in the words of Columbia Narrative Medicine.[211] The dietitian or nutritional professional can learn the power of listening to patient's stories for these deeper, existential needs. This allows Registered Dietitians to offer holistic care, in offering spiritual care inside of lifestyle medicine rather than engaging in conversation and support of VSED. VSED truncates the process of life reflection, which allows a person to formulate deeper meaning and a sense of purpose in living.

Also, even just reading about the PDQ interview done by another provider produced a significantly greater increase of compassion, a "knowledge of what others have faced in their lives which generated in the staff persons an empathetic response," and a "great deal of personal satisfaction" to know their patients as the people they are or were before the illness."[212]

Dignity-affirming care, although initially framed for palliative care, can truly impact medical care across the board, making the provider more aware of their own attitudes toward patients that may impact the care they provide. Rather than short-stepping care as described by promoting VSED, providers using dignity-affirming care can more often exhibit core values of kindness, respect, and dignity-promoting care consistent with the four premises of the Code of Ethics for the Nutrition and Dietetic Profession and the Hippocratic oath. The goal, according to Chochinov, is to "relocate humanity and kindness to their proper place in the culture of patient care," which "embraces the very essence of medicine."[213]

In complex times, practicing morally right, ethical care can be difficult and confusing. In the words of Salmasy from 2006, "The spirituality of medical practice at the dawn of the 21st Century [and in today's time] demands great virtue-courage, hope, perseverance, and creative fidelity."[214]

To go deeper, as a Registered Dietitian, consider the PDQ question for yourself. The goal is to reflect and decipher your own value system and manner of renewing your own human spirit, the essence of offering spiritual care inside of lifestyle medicine. Ask yourself, "What do I know about myself? What are my own challenges that I could share with others so they know me better?" When you approach your own medical provider, consider, "What do I want them to know about me as a person so they can give me the best care?" Ethical care is care that affirms the dignity of the person, which affirms their autonomy. It is built on working to provide care that does no harm but is further addressed by knowing them more deeply as people. Ethical care is built on trust, compassion, empathy, and learning about the human situation of those we care for.

To take the Patient Dignity Inventory, go to: https://dignityincare.ca/en/the-patient-dignity-inventory.html

# CHAPTER 9

*Understanding World Religious*

*Practices & Fasting*

Having a basic cultural competency to understand the basic tenets of different world religions is important, as "religion and spirituality are important factors in the majority of patients seeking care."[215] Religion and spirituality can impact eating or dietary practices, choices for medical care like blood transfusions, organ donation, autopsy, if religion can be a source for healing, which practices are prohibited (abortion, euthanasia, artificial insemination), rituals around death, pregnancy, if surgery is allowed, and the sex of the clinician providing care. Different religions have distinct parameters for practicing religious rituals, prayers, and symbols.

The following is a summary of major world religions, their basic tenets, and the influence of religious beliefs on death, diet, pregnancy, and practitioner relationships, along with considerations regarding fasting. This information aims to help practitioners better understand cultural parameters and effectively support, engage, and treat patients from diverse faith traditions. It is summarized from Swihart (2024) and the American Medical Association.

## Baha'i

Baha'i promotes the essential value, equality, and unity of all people and holds the goal of abandoning all prejudice: "race, religion, gender, or community." Each person is encouraged to seek truth, find oneness with God, to avoid extremes of poverty and wealth, and equality between the sexes to promote world peace. This faith considers a person's existence is spiritual and not physical.

Eating is practiced to promote health, and drugs are to be avoided if health is good but taken only when prescribed by a clinician and necessary to restore health. Members over age 15 are asked to fast from food and drink from sunrise to sunset during the month of Ala, March 2–20.

Blood transfusions and organ donation are allowed. After death, the body may not be transported more than one hour's journey from the place of death and should be buried, not cremated, preferably without embalming. Adherents rarely use birth control, do not believe in abortion, and only consider sexual intercourse between husband and wife acceptable. Participants are to practice daily prayer and have the nine-pointed star as a "symbol of faith."

# Buddhism

Buddhists follow diverse beliefs and practices stemming from the original teachings of Siddhartha Gautama, the Buddha. There are three prominent Buddhist traditions: Mahayana, Theravada, and Tibetan. Spiritual enlightenment, found through conscious living and meditation, replaces belief in God.

Buddhists typically seek holistic health, follow vegetarianism, and avoid alcohol, coffee, and tobacco. They also aim to avoid mind-altering drugs, as the state of mind during death impacts rebirth into the next life. They do not believe that healing comes through prayer or faith but arises from being awakened to the wisdom of the Buddha.

Buddhists believe that illness results from karma, which is the law of cause and effect stemming from a person's own actions. There are no restrictions on blood transfusions, organ donation, or medical procedures, and all medications are allowed as long as they do not affect consciousness or state of mind. Artificial insemination and birth control are acceptable, but abortion and the taking of life are not.

Adherents are encouraged to practice daily chanting and meditation, ordain both men and women, burn incense, and make offerings of fruit and flowers. They also have statues of Buddha, prayer beads, and chant boxes.

# Church of Jesus Christ of Latter-day Saints (Mormons)

Mormons are described as a movement of Restorationist Christianity that was started by Joseph Smith. Their beliefs center around the temple, where participants make personal and sacred covenants with the Lord. Jesus Christ is considered the firstborn of God, and all members are spiritual daughters and sons of a living Father in Heaven.

Autopsies, blood transfusions, and organ donations are allowed, while abortion and euthanasia are not. The belief is that all individuals who are part of this faith will be resurrected and obtain a degree of glory in heaven based on their actions during their lives. Procreation is viewed as a central purpose of life, and the decision to use birth control is left up to the couple.

Two elders are required to bless the sick, while designated leaders are called bishops and elders.

# Hinduism

This is one of the most ancient religions, dating back 4,000 years, and the third largest group with one billion followers worldwide. Adherents believe they hold the duty to "God, parents, society and teachers" and that promotes the goal to be freed from an imperfect world and reunite with God. Pain, suffering, and illness are the result of their prior actions (karma), and one's future life can be impacted by the way one faces disability, illness, or death with the goal of being reincarnated.

As a person is dying, the atmosphere must be calm and peaceful and immediately after death the "family may wash the body and the priest may pour water into the mouth." Most prefer to die at home and be cremated on the day of the death, although children under age two are buried.

Euthanasia is forbidden but there is no prohibition against clinical treatments or blood transfusions. They are against abortion.

Prayers for health are frowned upon as "stoicism is preferred." Women are not to express desires for special care, and all questions should be directed to the father or husband, who is considered the primary spokesperson for the family. Most are vegetarian or they may avoid beef and pork. The right hand is used for eating and the left for hygiene, bathing and toileting. Fasting is undertaken on certain days of the week in connection with certain deities, during special holy days and on certain days of the lunar calendar.

This is not a church-based religion and has no formal hierarchical structure. All participants in worship activities must sit at a lower elevation than the image of the deity and be barefoot. There are sacred objects present, such as candles, fresh flowers, incense, prayer beads, and sandalwood, along with sacred writings.

# Islam

Followers of Islam are called Muslims and believe in one God, Allah. They are guided by prophets including Abraham, David, Jesus, Moses, Noah, and Adam, as well as the Quran, which contains significant portions of the Bible's Old Testament. Muslims consider Muhammad to be God's messenger. He lived from 570 to 632 AD in Saudi Arabia. They seek complete submission to God, pray five times a day, and strive for life after death. Muslims are required to undertake a pilgrimage to Mecca at least once in their lifetime, give 2.5% of their income to charity each year, and observe a month-long fast during daylight hours in Ramadan. However, children, pregnant women, and those who are ill are exempt from fasting. Followers are encouraged to consume food that is "clean, good, pure, nourishing, pleasant, tasteful, and wholesome," but they must avoid vegetable oil, pork, shellfish and alcohol.

Autopsy is allowed only for legal or medical reasons. Euthanasia is prohibited. Organ donation, biopsies, blood, medications and amputations are allowed while most surgical procedures are allowed in addition. Abortion is prohibited.

Female patients typically require female care providers, and it is customary for handshakes or any contact between genders to be prohibited. Some women are required to wear a burqa or covering that includes the head, face, and entire body, including hands and feet. Others wear a hijab, or veil, that covers the head but not the face.

Fridays are the holy days for Muslims, marked by the Celebration of the Sacrifice of Abraham (Eid al-Adha), which is a three-day celebration, as well as the Celebration of Fast-breaking, among additional holy days.

## Judaism

Judaism is an ancient faith that expresses the covenant established by God with the Children of Israel. Although there are different sects of Judaism—Orthodox, Conservative, and Reform—all believe in one all-powerful God who created the universe, gave Moses the Torah on Mount Sinai, and established commandments, commitments, and duties. The books of the Torah are considered divine and are the source for following the "Code of Jewish Law," though interpretations vary from Orthodox to Reform.

Autopsy, organ donation, and blood products are acceptable, while cremation is discouraged or prohibited. Abortion is permitted only to save the life of the mother, and amputated limbs must be buried in consecrated ground. Some adherents may only consume Kosher food, food described in Jewish dietary laws determining how food is prepared and processed, although fish or fish/meat mix are not Kosher. A rabbi or religious leader may need to be consulted in reference to life-support or tube feeding. The feast of Purim is preceded by the Fast of Esther with no eating or drinking. There is also fasting on the Day of Atonement, Yom Kippur.

# Roman Catholicism

This is the oldest and largest Christian faith group worldwide. It believes that Jesus Christ founded it and is structured with hierarchical institutions starting from the original followers/apostles of Jesus. At this point, leaders are males organized by the Pope as the successor to Apostle Peter. There is emphasis on seven Sacraments that are visible signs of spiritual realities, including Baptism, Confession, Confirmation, Eucharist, Holy Orders, Prayers for the Sick, and Marriage.

Autopsy, organ donation, and blood products are allowed, while abortion and artificial birth control are prohibited. However, the Church supports couples in managing family size using the Symptothermal method or natural family planning. Fasting is encouraged on Good Friday and Ash Wednesday, and followers are asked to avoid meat on Fridays, especially during Lent (the 40 days prior to Easter), although fish is permitted. Aside from this, there are no strict dietary guidelines, but fasting for one hour prior to Mass and receiving the Eucharist is required. Those who are seriously ill or nearing death can request the presence of an ordained priest to administer the Sacrament of Anointing of the Sick. The Eucharist may be offered to individuals close to death if they can swallow. Concrete symbols often accompany prayer and sacred rituals; these include blessed holy water, prayer beads or Rosary beads, and lighting candles to symbolize requests for prayers. Bible texts from both the Old and New Testaments are compiled and used in all worship services as well as in many private devotions.

# Protestant Christians
(Amish, Anglican, Baptist, Christian, Churches of Christ,
Disciples of Christ, Episcopalian, Lutheran, Mennonites, Methodist,
Presbyterian and United Church of Christ)

Protestant Christians are followers of Christ who separated from Roman Catholicism as part of the Reformation movement. They emphasize justification by faith alone rather than by good works. Their beliefs and practices are grounded in the Bible, which serves as their source of faith and morals. Adherents value daily prayer and regularly gathering for community worship. They profess belief in two sacraments: Baptism and Communion, as ways to follow Jesus as the Savior of the world. Some denominations practice infant baptism and have other rituals, such as anointing. Participants believe in the power of prayer for healing.

There are no dietary restrictions or prohibitions on autopsy, receiving blood, or other clinical issues affecting healthcare. Euthanasia is generally not permissible, and birth control and artificial insemination are regarded as personal choices.

## Jehovah's Witness

Followers of Jehovah through Jesus Christ are a cohesive group who believe in the imminent destruction of the present world in order to usher in a restored state of paradise. In this way, followers of Christ will be resurrected with healthy physical bodies and inhabit the earth. They believe in "God as the Father, Jesus as the son and the Holy Spirit as God's motivating force," although they reject notions of the Holy Trinity. This group promotes adult baptism and shuns members who fail to live according to the group's principles.

Adherents consider organ donation and birth control a personal choice but consider euthanasia, abortion, artificial insemination by donors, eating food without draining out the blood prior to consumption and receiving any blood donation strictly prohibited.

## Seventh-day Adventist

This Protestant Christian group observes the Sabbath on Saturday, the seventh day of the week, and emphasizes the imminent Second Coming of Jesus Christ. Their teachings follow the Bible and align with the beliefs of other Protestant churches, including the Trinity and the inerrancy of the Bible. Adherents strive for holistic health, emphasizing a healthy diet and lifestyle, conservative principles, and the promotion of religious liberty. Practices such as autopsy, organ donation, receiving blood transfusions, and undergoing surgery, as well as using birth control, are permissible. They believe that "chaplains and physicians are inseparable," as the health of the body and the health of the soul are united. Religious leaders can be male or female, and ill individuals may be anointed with oil by elders or pastors. Participants generally follow a vegetarian diet, promote therapeutic diets, fast on occasion, and consider alcohol, coffee, and tea to be avoided.

## Spirituality—Hawaiian

This spirituality emphasizes oneness and connection to those who have departed this earth. Daily spiritual practices cultivate a sense of community with all natural things, unity with others, and self-greatness, which is known as developing the "aloha spirit." Wearing a lei in a complete circle is thought to ward off bad circumstances. There is no death, only a transition from human to spiritual form. Poor health is considered the result of not living in harmony with nature, as health and healthcare are intertwined with Hawaiian culture and religious beliefs. Health arises from the connection of the body, mind, and spirit. Fasting is a regular practice, but otherwise, there are no dietary restrictions or limits on medical treatments. Silence, observation, and respect for both male and female religious leaders are highly valued virtues. There are no sacred texts or writings, but stories are passed down orally. Fasting and ritual washing can precede ceremonial rituals where ho'okupu are offered.

## Spirituality—Native American

Native American spirituality and practices vary by tribe but share some common elements, including aspects of Hawaiian spirituality. Native spirituality centers around the fundamental interconnectedness of all natural things, such as life, land, and Mother Earth, and it promotes a strong sense of community. The terms "God" and "Creator" are used interchangeably. Poor health is believed to result from a failure to live in harmony with nature, as well as social and supernatural environments. There are no dietary restrictions or issues affecting surgery, clinical practice, or receiving blood. Prayer, which often involves sacred objects and the burning of cedar, sage, sweetgrass, or tobacco, aims to enhance one's ability to see and understand a vision more clearly for oneself.

## Common Fasting Practices

Fasting, which is the voluntary abstention from food and drink, is linked to several physical benefits. These include reductions in mTor,[216] chronic inflammation, cardiovascular disease (CVD) risk factors, and insulin resistance, contributing to better metabolic health, provided no eating disorders are present.[217]

For many people, fasting is an essential path to spiritual purification. Various religions advocate fasting for its spiritual benefits, often minimizing food intake during specific seasons. For instance, many Christians observe Lent, a 40-day period before Easter, while Muslims engage in Ramadan, a 28–30-day annual period of modified fasting that shifts with the Islamic calendar each year. Buddhists typically promote fasting six days a month by refraining from food from noon until dawn as a means to cultivate spiritual growth through self-mastery.

## Muslim eating practices218

Food, according to Laws outlined in the Quran, has important spiritual value. Many eating practices follow the statues from the Prophet Mohammad who lived 570–632 AD. Olives, honey, yogurt, dates, figs, grapes, pomegranates, and legumes are important components of Muslim eating practices. According to Islamic law, all foods are considered lawful or *halal* except for pork and its by-products, animals improperly slaughtered or dead before slaughtering, animals slaughtered in the name of anyone but Allah (God), carnivorous animals, birds of prey, animals without externals ears (some bird and reptiles), blood, alcohol and foods contaminated with any of these. Seafood is lawful. The Islamic Food and Nutrition Council of America offers a certification to label foods free of the offending foods.

Many Muslims are avid label readers to ascertain whether foods contain by-products of offending foods like gelatin, emulsifiers and enzymes.

## Muslim fasting practices

During Ramadan, Muslims, according to Islamic Law, are asked not to consume all foods and drinks, including water and gum, from sun up to sun down. Fasting is a "pillar of the religion and a highly valued act of worship." The primary spiritual benefits of fasting, according to Muslims, are that it brings spiritual peace and intensifies worship of God. Commonly, Islamic persons attempt to consume nutrient-dense foods that detoxify the body.

The two main meals of the day are suhur (immediately prior to dawn) and iftar (just after sunset), mealtimes that coincide with two of the five times of daily prayer. For suhur, foods typically eaten for dinner, or leftovers or ethnic foods are consumed. Dates and a cup of water are common foods eaten to break the fast at the end of the day.

During certain situations, Muslims are exempt from fasting: travel, menstruation, illness or older age, pregnancy, and breastfeeding. With medical conditions, especially diabetes, heart disease, kidney disease and peptic ulcers, patients most often desire to comply with fasting routines, so care plans with eating and medication have to be tailored to fasting periods.

## Buddhist eating practices

While there are several forms of Buddhism each with distinct dietary practices, all Buddhists attempt to follow the practices of Buddha from the 4th and 5th centuries BC. Buddha prohibits taking the life of any person or animal so most Buddhists avoid eating meat, fish, poultry and eggs although they consume dairy products. Some consume meat as long as it is not slaughtered primarily for them. Laws prohibit consuming excessive alcohol to avoid clouding the mind or strong-smelling vegetables like garlic, onions, and chives, as they are thought to increase sexual desire when cooked or anger when eaten raw.

## Hindu fasting and feasting practices[219]

The honorable Supreme Court of India defines Hinduism as a way of life rather than a religion. "Hindu" refers to a group of people who adhere to the supremacy of the Vedas and follow certain prescribed paths for living. These followers are called Sruti. Fasting can involve various practices: nirahara (complete fasting), phalahara (fasting with fruit and milk), or alpahara (allowing broken rice, as intact rice is prohibited during this period). Eating practices alternate between periodic fasting on certain days of the week and feasting or fasting during festivals. The specific days designated as fast days and the timing of festivals vary among different sects of Hinduism.

## Fasting for Catholics

For the Latin Church, members aged 18 to 59 are asked to fast on Ash Wednesday, the first Wednesday marking the beginning of Lent, and on Good Friday, the Friday of Holy Week before Easter. They should also fast one hour before receiving the Eucharist at Mass. The dates of Lent and Easter vary based on the lunar cycle, specifically the first full moon following the spring equinox.

Members of the Eastern Catholic Church follow their own sui iuris Church regulations, which are specific to their community. These rules often coincide with those of the Latin Church. During fasting, individuals may consume one main meal per day along with two smaller meals, which together should not equal the size of the main meal. Fasting is intended to promote self-management, enhance healthy self-denial, and improve one's ability to pray. Participants are also asked to abstain from meat during Fridays in Lent, as well as on Ash Wednesday and Good Friday.

## Fasting for Greek Orthodox[220]

Members of the Greek Orthodox Church fast for 180 to 200 days each year. Their primary fasting periods include the Nativity Fast (40 days before Christmas), Lent (48 days before Easter), and the Assumption Fast (15 days in August). Fasters follow a vegetarian diet, primarily abstaining from dairy products, eggs, and meat every day, while also avoiding fish and olive oil on Wednesdays and Fridays. During the rest of the year, adherents are encouraged to fast similarly on Wednesdays and Fridays, except for the days following Christmas, Easter, and Pentecost. It is interesting to note that daily calorie intake may vary during these fasting periods, as Greek Orthodox Christians often increase their carbohydrate intake and decrease their fat intake during this time.[221]

## Christian Daniel Fast[222]

This fast is based on the story from the Book of Daniel, in which Daniel vowed not to defile himself with royal food and drink and to eat only vegetables (pulses) and water for 10 days. Modern Daniel fasts allow adherents to eat foods ad libitum, but the food choices are restricted to fruits, vegetables, whole grains, legumes, nuts, seeds, and oil, similar to the vegan pattern. This fast focuses on whole foods and prohibits processed foods and sweets

# CHAPTER 10

*How Does Growing in Spiritual*

*Sensitivity Help Prevent Burnout*

*for the Dietitian?*

"Spirituality is thus understood as an important skill, gained through experience, a lingua franca which enables health practitioners to communicate around important matters."[223] Clinicians become more skilled in communicating about spiritual needs as they gain "spiritual skills" from working with patients. As we have been discussing, to notice these spiritual themes in their patients' lives and narratives, clinicians must develop greater sensitivity to the spiritual dimensions of their own lives. In the second section of this resource, we will elaborate in more detail on the skills that help dietitians develop this spiritual sensitivity and the capacity to offer spiritual care to people from diverse spiritual perspectives and cultures. To start, in addition to what you have already done, consider filling out one of the spiritual assessment tools from the Appendix. Reflect on what is true for you in your own life, slow down, and use the insights that arise while completing the spiritual assessment tools. Pay attention to your feelings, questions, insights, and moments of awe as you go about your day. Intentionally spend time in nature, do something creative, listen to music, pray, or meditate. Allow this process of cultivating spiritual attentiveness to guide your awareness as you respond to the events in your own life and the lives of your clients.

Whether you possess a religious faith or if you are an agnostic or atheist, do any of these descriptions of spirituality touch or move you? Pay attention to your subjective reactions in the discussion and how you have seen spirituality impact your life or those around you. It's just like the wind; you can't see it, but you feel it on your cheek. Are any of these ideas of spirituality practical means by which you could deepen your own spirituality? I am inviting you, even if you have a long-standing religious faith, to review the checklist that describes spirituality in Chapter 3, and the discussions that follow, and consider how something new can deepen what you already experience. Look and listen with fresh eyes. Be open and avoid the common temptation we discussed in the Preface to maintain the "status quo" of what you've always known. You want to build upon it and deepen your spirituality! Remember that spirituality and religious faith are dynamic! By reflecting on what you've always believed, you come to understand life differently.

One night, as I was writing this, I glanced at the alarm clock on my bedside table and wondered how old it was. Unlike my husband, who had switched to using his cell phone as an alarm, I still relied on this little white box with the radio. It had been my trusted companion and had woken me up for longer than I could remember. I asked aloud, "When did I get this thing?" Determined, I rummaged through the other room for my cell phone, even though it was past my bedtime. I found information about it in what I playfully called the "alarm clock museum." I bought it a year after passing the RD exam, at the start of my career, over 35 years ago! I had looked at that clock face while timing my contractions in the middle of the night with my first baby, the morning we flew to Europe, the day each of my six kids graduated from high school, and the night I received the call that my mother's condition had worsened and she was dying. This clock represented my life in review. Today, I encourage you to examine your faith or spiritual expression, just as I did with my trusted alarm clock. Investigate it, appreciate it, and consider adding something new and alive in gratitude for all the ways this essence has accompanied you throughout your life, allowing it to grow within you.

Practitioners best develop the capacity to recognize spiritual movements and resources in another, by keying into their own spirituality and human foibles to grow in sensitivity. Consider your own life and see if your need for perfection or absolute security, or the loss of clarity of your mission, or anything else is fragmenting you. Also, listen for and notice what is missing in the lives of your clients. As you work with them, consider what they most need from you emotionally and from your evidence-based wheelhouse.

What we are after is to grow our sensitivity and our savvy so we can help ourselves and our clients more holistically to build their health and well-being. We want to highlight the light and personal efficacy that can spring forth in our lives when we grow in our awareness of spirituality. Find some encouragement for this from a poem from Seamus Heaney (2010), a Nobel-prize poet who illustrates the importance of opening our eyes and clearing our senses to spiritual realities.

> *Had I not been awake I would have missed it,*
> *A wind that rose and whirled until the roof*
> *Pattered with quick leaves off the sycamore*
> *And got me up, the whole of me a-patter,*
> *Alive and ticking like an electric fence:*

## Positive self-care for nutritionists and dietitians

Besides just assisting clients to cultivate lives of meaning and purpose and to deal with spiritual distress and grief in a way that renews their human spirits, spiritual care is something that practitioners can apply to caring for themselves. Dietitians are practitioners who care deeply about people. In fact, empathy, the capacity to "appreciate, to effectively communicate an understanding of the patient's experiences and perspectives,"[225] is a "key skill for dietitians" and lifestyle medicine providers to develop in clinical practice. But, do clinicians extend this same skill and call for "lifelong learning" in empathy to having compassion toward themselves?

An even more interesting reflection to consider are the words of Salmasy, "The work of all healthcare professionals is fraught with deeper meaning than they often realize. It is the profound mystery of the person that stirs- not just blood but life." Do lifestyle medicine providers slow down and consider this mystery for themselves to renew their own storehouse?

Studies show that empathy is malleable. Clinicians can learn and grow in empathy "by experience and education or *lose it* through neglect, desensitization, and burnout."[226] Being empathetic towards others is a prime way dietitians often engage in spiritual care without knowing that's what they are doing.

 In a large study, 8,038 dietitians were surveyed to assess their job satisfaction, degree of burnout and level of emotional intelligence. Of those, 89.1% of dietitians surveyed had strong emotional intelligence. Interestingly, emotional intelligence correlated positively with both job satisfaction and, eventually, with burnout.[227] It seems that people who care a lot and have high EI to notice others' pain can easily move from a satisfying level of compassion to compassion fatigue. This impacts emotional, physical and spiritual health negatively. Would growing spiritual intelligence counter this tendency to burnout?

What seems to be missing for the practitioner who is burning out is a pattern and tempo of regular self-care and self-awareness that allows them to stay in touch with their "divine spark" or human essence. Learning spiritual care for the dietitian takes on a new light. When practitioners mature in their spiritual awareness, they more easily can recognize their own needs and what can renew them as well as what motivates them to follow through with self-care reflection and activities before they burn out.

Until now, the discussion about self-care activities for practitioners has focused on the specifics of what to do for good self-care rather than developing spirituality that animates and deepens commitment to self-care and active self-awareness. Practitioners have missed the human formation that helps them interpret pain, suffering, vocation, meaning/purpose that can help form personal margins and perspective when they encounter pain and suffering in their patients.

"The risks come," as one therapist stated, "from getting perilously close to the flame that burns deep within the sorrow of each client that we see."[228] This rather frequent exposure to pain and suffering can bring emotional exhaustion, even numbness for some, leaving a majority of RDs and healthcare professionals feeling underprepared for witnessing stories of trauma, pain, and suffering.[229] The good news is that "empathy in nutrition and dietetics can be taught and improved irrespective of career state."[230]

Team this with having a stressful and demanding job where they often are exposed to suffering, ethical issues, stress and sometimes feelings of not being respected in their jobs, it makes sense that they may be dealing with a tendency to burn out according to Dr. Gandotra.[231] Dr Gandotra continues, "Most importantly, they (dietitians) are often expected to come in to fix the problem with a patient. But there's a lot more at play in helping a patient become healthy." Maybe that's why when Career Explorer surveyed dietitians in the USA, they found low job satisfaction among them.[232] Dietitians rated their job satisfaction 2.9 out of a possible 5, putting them in the bottom 26% of all professions for fulfillment on the job. Nutritional professionals can admit their vulnerabilities and learn new skills to "fan the spark into a flame."

As a profession, science and evidence have been the focus of the training in both academic and clinical practicum education. In an insightful dissertation, Honig[233] notes an important omission, stating, for example, "ASCEND, Accreditation Council for Education in Nutrition and Dietetics, does not require nutrition and dietetics programs to address compassion fatigue (or spiritual care) in the required courses."

Some training programs for student dietitians, however, show signs of noticing this need for skills to sustain well-being among nutritional professionals. For example, Griffith University in Australia instituted the "Resilience and Well-being Program" for 111 dietetic students for 6 weeks in the first trimester of the third year of training, prior to the practicum. The hope was to train dietetic students in stress management, coping strategies, and self-care, which include how to recognize emotions in themselves in the practice of meditation, with strategies to form better life-work balance. Ninety-nine percent felt that it was helpful and allowed them to implement more positive lifestyle behaviors, have a more balanced life, better self-regulation, and a more positive mindset.[234] This effort appears to support students in finding the common thread or coherence in living that helped them "recover, adapt, and grow from a challenge."[235] This type of training while still in school has not been the norm for most nutritional professionals trained in the USA.

Research has shown that spiritual care training and support of spiritual identities improve practitioners' spiritual health and reduce work-related stress and burnout.[236] In fact, among nurses caring for critically ill Covid-19 patients during the pandemic, those with stronger religious or spiritual identities showed growth in spiritual well-being even when exposed to traumatic events in "risking their own health and life, contact with patient's suffering or death." This shows that valuing "healthcare personnel's cultural and religious identity and encouraging self-reflective activities, such as mindfulness and meditation as well as religious practice can help to promote post-traumatic growth."[237] Can this be food for thought for training programs for dietitians, or professional development programs, or even for managers who supervise clinicians?

In fact, nutritional and lifestyle medicine professionals who manage other healthcare employees carry the responsibility to consider and grow in their own connection to spirituality. Research shows that when managers have "spiritual intelligence" or are spiritually sensitive, they are able to exercise a more "refined awareness of the present situation" in their responsibility and are better able to organize the practices to prevent compassion fatigue in those under them.[238] Managers with better spiritual intelligence also become more able to prioritize goals and allow situations to guide them, which encourages a better sense of mutual trust between directors and employees.[239]

## Personal Reflection Activity

Consider what would support your connection to the divine, the transcendent: Plan a time of prayer, creativity, and community connection that helps you cultivate peacefulness and grow spiritually. If you feel moved, read the Loving Kindness Nourishment Meditation and notice what surfaces in your own reflections.

Sometimes using a structured instrument (spiritual assessment tool) with a client for a time or two can help you also internalize what is involved in assessing someone's spiritual needs. They can fill it out with onboarding forms or this can serve as a guide you read over to remember what to look for in noticing spiritual needs. Spiritual assessments can also help us recognize in the moment something spiritual in our own experiences. If we notice that we felt deep peace when we walked outside and let our minds go or when we practiced meditation or centering prayer, we can return to it the next day and go deeper.

## Loving Kindness Nourishment Meditation

As you consider your own responses or reflect on situations with your patients, consider if you could suggest using something like this Loving Kindness Nourishment Meditation to provide spiritual care inside your disciple and promote healing of body and soul. Read it slowly, then imagine the words touching you. Quiet your breathing and your sympathetic nervous system. Notice if it has any lasting effects. Remember, spirituality is more than something that is defined; it is a dimension of living.

Anyone can practice this meditation on loving kindness, whether they are religious or not. It is a practice and a technique.

The aim of this meditation is to find what we are deeply hoping to experience in our lives. We can start with a suggested phrase but notice what our heart/mind most desires and adjust it accordingly.

As we attempt this reflection, we need to slow down, notice the present moment and let ourselves rest in this process. Surprising results can happen if we do! This is a 3-minute meditation.

You can start by taking delight in your own goodness—calling to mind things you have done out of good-heartedness, and rejoice in those memories. We celebrate the potential for goodness we all share.

**Consider your body, that you are wonderfully made** and at any given moment your heart is beating and pumping blood through blood vessels and can sync with the music and sounds you hear. Your nose picks up 1 trillion smells. You have a unique fingerprint and tongue pattern. Your body carries you.

**Think about nourishing your body with love, to provide care, nurture, energize and calm** your cells which make you. Think about providing enough water, energy, building blocks and nutrients.

**Pray or open the door for your body to receive goodness.** Rest in the goodness of your body and your health.

Consider your smile, the first expression babies learn and a sign of happiness and good will.

**Smile at yourself and consider your goodness.** Enjoy the taste of your favorite foods and imagine them providing nutrition to your amazing body. What is one thing that you wish for yourself?

**Silently recite phrases that reflect what you wish most** deeply for yourself.

- May I have peace and joy.
- May life make me whole, or healthy.
- May I live with ease or have light to see.

**Visualize yourself in the center of a circle composed of those who have been kind to you,** or have inspired you because of their love. Keep gently repeating the phrases of loving kindness for yourself.

**To close the session, let go of the visualization.** Keep reflecting that you are nourishing yourself, and are moving forward, sustained by the force of kindness.

## Personal Reflection Activity

When we ask ourselves important or "lofty questions," we often grow more relaxed, more focused, and aware of our needs, hopes, assets, and desires. They promote a mind shift from the negative to the positive and help us consider new possibilities for ourselves and those we work with. Write your responses down.

- What am I most passionate about in living and in my practice?
- What fears are holding me back and how can I confront these?
- What am I most grateful for today and why?
- Ask yourself what is the most significant concern or emotion that the patient is experiencing?
- Did you notice any grief issues or issues of distress from what you know?
- How did you address this spiritually impactful experience in the midst of nutrition counseling?

Use one of the following spiritual assessment scales to experiment learning new aspects of spirituality in your own life or in the lives of your clients. Maybe you have never considered something spiritual when, in fact, it is. Assessing yourself for signs and symptoms of carried grief can be helpful for you in caring for your soul or human-divine spark.

## Spiritual Well-Being Scale

**We are trying to awaken greater sensitivity to our daily experiences. See if this inventory helps you be more alert this week to spiritual experiences in your own life.**

**Answer 1=Strongly agree, 2=Agree, 3=Neither agree nor disagree, 4= Disagree, 5= Strongly Disagree**

1. I don't find much satisfaction in private prayer with God/Higher Power or spiritual meditation.

2. I don't know who I am, where I came from or where I am going.

3. I believe that God/HP or the positive force of the Universe loves me and cares about me.

4. I feel that life is a positive experience.

5. I believe that God/HP or a Force is impersonal and not interested in my daily situation.

6. I feel unsettled about my future.

7. I have a personally meaningful relationship with God/HP or Force of the Universe.

8. I feel very fulfilled and satisfied with life.

9. I don't get much personal strength and support from my God/HP or spirituality.

10. I feel a sense of well-being about the direction my life is headed.

11. I believe that God/HP or the Force of the Universe is concerned about my problems.

12. I don't enjoy much about life.

13. I don't have a personally satisfying relationship with God/HP or my spirituality.

14. I feel good about my future.

15. My relationship with God/HP or the Universe helps me not to feel lonely.

16. I feel that life is full of conflict and unhappiness.

17. I feel most fulfilled when I'm in close communion with God/HP or my spirituality.

18. Life doesn't have much meaning.

19. My relation with God/HP or the Force of the Universe contributes to my sense of well-being.

20. I believe there is some real purpose for my life.

**Add up your score. Scores 10–20= a mod/poor relationship with God, 21–49 = moderate satisfying relationship with God, 50-60=positive relationship with God/HP**

## Additional Spiritual Assessment Tools

**Spiritual Care Self-Assessment Tool**

1.  I have a way of thinking (or a way of believing) that supports or builds me up. YES. NO If Yes: The name or a description of my thinking/believing/ spirituality/philosophy/religion is:

    _____

2.  The influence of my THINKING and PRACTICES on the way I care for myself is:

    _____

3.  There is conflict between my THINKING and PRACTICES and the medical situation/care/decision-making that I face. YES or NO, If Yes: the Conflict is:

    _____

**Check off any of the following statements that are true:**

○   I am having doubts about my thinking/faith/beliefs/practices

○   I am in conflict with my faith/spiritual community and/or its leadership

○   I am not sure what I believe anymore

○   I somehow keep doing other than what I know I out to be doing

○   I feel guilty about the way I think, feel or act

○   It sometimes seems to me like I am being punished

○   I feel angry for what is happening to me

○   I feel alone.

○   It feels to me like I've let someone or something down

○   I wrestle with whether or not I measure up and am loved

○   I sometimes think that evil is involved here, somehow.

○   I sometimes ask, "Why?" or, in other words,

     "What is the meaning or purpose of this medical situation?

**There are months when I have difficulty making ends meet.**

| 1. | 2. | 3. | 4. | 5 |
|---|---|---|---|---|
| Not at all. | Rarely. | More than a bit. | Fairly often. | Always |

I am struggling to cope.

| 1. | 2. | 3. | 4. | 5 |
|---|---|---|---|---|
| Not at all. | Rarely. | More than a bit. | Fairly often. | Always |

I have people who care about me.

| 1. | 2. | 3. | 4. | 5 |
|---|---|---|---|---|
| Not at all. | Rarely. | More than a bit. | Fairly often. | Always |

People who support me.　　　What they do to help me.　　Conflicts I have

**What I hold onto in difficult times (what sustains me and keeps me going) is:**

The practices that I use to build myself up are:

Check all that apply

O  Music (playing, singing, listening)

O  Crafts (knitting, sewing, shop, etc.)

O  Walking

O  Attention to diet

O  Communing with nature

O  Pet care

O  Study

O  Prayer

O  Other

O  Art (creation, appreciation)

O  Job/work/vocation

O  Physical activity/workout

O  Substance use (cigarettes, alcohol, drugs)

O  Gardening

O  Leisure reading

O  Devotional reading

O  Attending religious services

O  Relationships within faith, culture, or neighborhood community

On the same level above, mark routines that are missing for you right now.

**I worry there are practices I use to cope which may be harmful or destructive:**

YES or NO

# In summary of the first portion of this work

As the first portion of this work culminates, we hope that you have come to a new realization of the call for dietitians and lifestyle medicine practitioners to integrate spiritual care inside of the care process. In many ways, this is a call to just claim some of the things that dietitians and other providers have already found themselves doing in the midst of providing compassionate and empathetic care to their patients. The professional's goal is often to discuss food intake and macronutrients, but patients usually trust RDs and providers so they share what else is also on their minds and in their hearts. They may cry when they receive the results of food sensitivity testing when they see that their favorite foods are causing a reaction, and they recount all the memories of eating that food with people who might be gone. Dietitians inadvertently catch clients in the midst of life, grief, and discouragement associated with changing long-standing habits or giving up habits that have helped them cope with the ups and downs of life—the seeming nurturing from sweets, etc.

Many times, when these deeply held issues come up, practitioners have struggled to have their bearings about what to say and what these issues are tied to. Often, these issues poke places inside the practitioner that the practitioner did not know were there and that are festering. Such are the gifts and graces of working closely in collaboration with patients. Practitioners struggle not to be overwhelmed with secondary trauma as patients dump their stories in the midst of the session. Sometimes, it is hard to know how to leave work at work, and the practitioner feels burdened and forever changed by knowing what they know.

The aim here is to present the growing evidence that spirituality affects health and well-being. To practice whole-person care effectively, practitioners need training to learn how to focus their empathy to help clients and care for themselves. Positive spirituality serves as a resource for both clinicians and patients, while prolonged spiritual distress and grief can have physical effects on the body. Until now, nutrition professionals may not have known how to leverage spirituality as a resource for health. Many might have assumed this exploration was purely religious. It is important to note that spirituality and religion are distinct; however, they can exist separately or integrate within a person's life.

Some dietitians are "fixers" who get called in to be people in the know, when research shows that patients generally want the *fixer* to morph into a *collaborative and warm caregiver* who really knows and cares about them.[240] Generally, most dietitians try to be that, but many times at a cost to themselves personally, for it can be depleting. To provide this therapeutic practice while remaining the objective clinician who cares, dietitians must develop skills and tools to help companion clients into a healthy, well-lived life. This does not mean that your skills are deficient but only that you can deepen them and direct them differently with professional education and support in spiritual care training. These tools and skills will be the focus of the next portion of the text.

The goal is to present this provocative vision and a means to accomplish it. In the second portion of this work, we attempt to weave meaningful activities and situations so you can integrate them into your daily life and clinical practice.

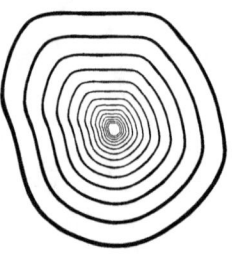

# PART
# 2

# CHAPTER 11

*Getting to the Heart of it: What Dietitians Offer to Spiritual Care that Is Unique and Has Been Missing*

In summarizing the previous discussion and cited research, spirituality is a positive health asset that, when cultivated, motivates people to more readily adopt positive health behaviors that can diminish inflammation, which exacerbates many chronic metabolic, cardiovascular, and mental health issues. On the flip side, patients stuck in spiritual distress and grief often experience a greater likelihood of having stress negatively impacting the cardiovascular and nervous systems and metabolism and more often present with glucose-regulation problems. Grieving people more frequently struggle with self-care and eating practices with food, gravitating more often to highly processed comfort foods, which they show a stronger negative physiological response to than non-grieving people.

However, proper spiritual support from practitioners (which will be explained in this next session) that, in a nutshell, includes listening to their feelings and narratives, providing perspectives of hope, helping connect them to spiritual practices, community support and further insight into their own vocations, allows the practitioner to stay emotionally available to accompany clients to address deeper issues that impact well-being and health.[241] This hopefully renews the client and clinician's human spirits as part of lifestyle medicine. Clients, hopefully, more readily move forward to live lives with greater meaning, purpose, resiliency, and physical health with this holistic care. Dietitians' unique emphasis on "health vitality" and wellness, as well as their skills in medical nutrition therapy to address disease states, allows the field to present a balanced and innovative view of spiritual care. Until now, this novel contribution to spiritual care inside of healthcare from dietitians and nutritionists, and principally a mode of training dietitians in spiritual care, has not been described in the literature from this author's inquiry. Lifestyle medicine has been missing the contribution that dietitians and providers can make when they include spiritual assessment and spiritual care to rebalance the lifestyle.

If spiritual care, then, offers so many benefits to achieving a healthy lifestyle and well-lived lives, what has stopped practitioners from being effective in offering spiritual care? The considerations are many. There is much confusion and a diversity of understandings about spiritual care as it is included in healthcare and how to train practitioners to offer it. Perspectives from nursing literature show that nursing struggles to identify, define, and assess spirituality and spiritual care within the healthcare relationship.[242] The Europe EPPICC Project describes that "spiritual care is care which recognizes and responds to the human spirit when faced with life-changing events (birth, trauma, ill health, loss) or sadness and can include the need for meaning, for self-worth to express oneself, for faith support, perhaps for rites or prayer or sacrament or simply for a sensitive listener."[243] What is missing in this is what happens if patients want to utilize spiritual practices to be well when they are not struggling with loss, disease, or being disheartened. Is this still a request for spiritual care? Also, within healthcare, there seems to be no consensus on how to equip clinicians to address spiritual needs. Do practitioners want to develop the sensitivity this care requires on top of their technical skills?

Others describe taking "a broad perspective of spirituality" within nursing and state that spiritual care is learning "about the reality and nature of patients' spiritual needs and spiritual well-being in real-life situations," in the words of Baldacchino.[244] Baldacchino emphasizes being rather than simply doing, and the "therapeutic use of self" is of utmost importance. This perspective is so experiential that educators and practitioners alike may not know how this differs from psychological support or religious care from a pastor. Yet, in a recent scoping review of education interventions within nursing, Rykkje outlines, "Spiritual care is essential in caring for the whole person,"[245] which implies once again that spiritual care is an important aspect to consider for being well, maybe part of finding the life coherence of salutogenisis.

To remedy this confusion, educators within nursing principally have set competencies for spiritual care. Competence is considered "the proven ability to use knowledge, skills and personal, social and/or methodological abilities in the work or study situations and in professional and personal development," according to The Nursing and Midwifery Council in the UK in 2002.[246] According to this author and others,[247] developing competencies is just a starting place: to begin the investigation of including spirituality in holistic care but not a place to dwell, quibble, or become confused. To become competent in something, the person has to be formed on how to discerningly use the skills or competencies for different people.

Interestingly, too, if existential meaning, faith and spirituality grow and mature over time through stages,[248] which is true, the capacity to deliver spiritual care and how to train for it must also mature and grow through stages. In fact, clinicians being trained in spiritually infused care must be guided in how to keep growing and learning from life and professional care situations. Developing spiritual care competencies is the bare bones of where to start, but spiritual care is something more than a competency to measure, audit, or a task to check off.

Spirituality hits at the heart of the practice of dietetics and lifestyle medicine. Learning from Puchalski et al.[249] and the formation of physicians, this is seen in like fashion that "spirituality is the basis of their call as physicians and that spirituality is the basis of their compassionate relationship with their patients." She also says that in order "to express compassion and be present to another's suffering, they have to address their own spirituality in their lives." It is the same for dietitians and nutritionists. Considering spirituality in this way allows it to be protective for the practitioner and person alike and typically very impactful for the person receiving care.[250]

For example, in a small study at Harvard Medical School, fourth-year medical students who had higher scores for religion and spirituality showed greater ability to experience feelings and less tendency to repress feelings while caring for patients in difficult situations compared to the non-religious fourth-year medical students. They also showed less relational strife or competitive attitudes toward other students and better work-life balance.[251] Religious and spiritually oriented students observed that they became more religious during the study, largely due to their exposure to patient care. They found that their spirituality helped protect them from burnout and compassion fatigue. Clinicians also recognized the influence of spirituality on their lives after receiving support from divinity students in Clinical Pastoral Education. Additionally, they benefited from the modeling and mentoring of these students in how to have spiritual conversations.

Spirituality and faith, then, are developmental processes. They mature over time and follow charted paths of growth[252] in response to living and developing complex modes of practice.[253] [254] [255] This growth comes from training that supports understanding spirituality and applying spiritual care strategies in working with real people, as well as learning from one's own experiences and observing other practitioners' examples.[256] If this understanding is missed and spiritual care training is arranged as a one-shot assignment, a single class, or a short video series, practitioners remain hesitant and lack the confidence to offer spiritual support.[257] They also may attempt to listen and ask about religion or spirituality, but their attitudes remain fixed and they report "no increased ability to endure in situations without a solution or right answer"[258] or to endure in meaningless or powerless circumstances.

The capacity to offer spiritual care comes from seeing the learning process as something dynamic and experiential. It touches more than the intellect and hopefully activates the human spirit in such a way that the dietitian or lifestyle medicine practitioner can reach the very heart of what drew him or her to becoming a dietitian or healthcare professional to stay more grounded and see how they are uniquely equipped to offer healing care. In like fashion, this hard-earned awareness alerts them to their own needs, which they can more readily address before experiencing burnout and allowing them to blight their professional practice.

Caring for the human spirit helps dietitians grow in spiritual intelligence, enabling them to respond to their own thoughts and feelings as well as those of their patients. This growth allows clinicians to better meet patients' needs. Spiritual care involves more than just using spiritual language or discussing overtly religious issues. Training and support to develop spiritual intelligence promote their craft and wisdom in practice and prevent clinicians from avoiding necessary conversations due to discomfort.[259]

Some suggest that this philosophy of meeting spiritual needs within healthcare represents a "secular version of Judeo-Christian spirituality. Therefore, there is the potential for some faith traditions to be offended by the term (spirituality) as applied to healthcare."[260] To explore this question, it may be relevant to turn to a sacred scripture that was found to resonate from sacred texts from Judaism, Christianity, and Islam, and be reflected in Buddhism, to debunk this concern, to let "scripture's faith in divine potential of all human beings guide us."[261]

What hopefully happens when a person explores a sacred text is that they are moved from a simple cognitive awareness of truth to "areas of deepest meaning, which some might refer to as sacred, which underscores the importance of attending to their spiritual or inner life" (Puchalski & Guenther 2012). While the author knows that it may be difficult for readers from different faith traditions or from no faith tradition at all to feel comfortable reflecting on a sacred text from another culture, what is hoped is that readers find some common premises. Beauty attracts reflection. This may lead them to a new awareness that dynamic training in spiritual care comes from awakening competencies by reflecting on life and patient care experiences, with support that allows clinicians to mature to find deeper meaning, purpose, and connection to spirituality in living.

As an example, the following sacred words come both from Ezekiel 37:1-10 in Judeo-Christian Scripture and from the Qu'ran in Surah Al-Baqarah verse 245 and the Surah 'Abasa verse 27 and 36:78. Their essence is also reflected in Buddhist philosophy and the 4 Noble Truths: that humans become awakened in response to receiving transcendence and to quieting what distracts from recollection. Consider the following sacred text.

> The hand of the LORD came upon me, and he led me out in the spirit of the LORD and set me in the center of the broad valley. It was filled with bones. He made me walk among them in every direction. So many lay on the surface of the valley! How dry they were! He asked me: Son of man, can these bones come back to life? "Lord GOD," I answered, "you alone know that." Then he said to me: Prophesy over these bones, and say to them: Dry bones, hear the word of the LORD! Thus says the Lord GOD to these bones: Listen! I will make breath enter you so you may come to life. I will put sinews on you, make flesh grow over you, cover you with skin, and put breath into you so you may come to life. Then you shall know that I am the LORD.

> I prophesied as I had been commanded. A sound started up, as I was prophesying, rattling like thunder. The bones came together, bone joining to bone. As I watched, sinews appeared on them, flesh grew over them, skin covered them on top, but there was no breath in them.

> Then he said to me: Prophesy to the breath, prophesy, son of man! Say to the breath: Thus says the Lord GOD: From the four winds come, O breath, and breathe into these slain that they may come to life. I prophesied as he commanded me, and the breath entered them; they came to life and stood on their feet, a vast army.

Spiritual life or breath then draws the human person together, bones, sinew, and life. This force is received and active, forming new fullness, enlightenment, and spontaneous experiences in connecting with others and nature. Thus, humans are more than biological processes. The focus on competencies, spiritual assessment tools,on identifying clients with spiritual needs in order to apply specific modalities to meeting these needs become like "dry bones." In our thinking and what will be described later, spiritual care is something that has needed to be enfleshed and animated with a mode that breathes new breath into the discussion. Addressing spirituality is a dynamic process.

What's more, a healing therapeutic relationship is "bidirectional…and the clinical encounter *is* sacred" or carries the sense that something greater than oneself is active in the clinical encounter and "poignant or perhaps moving."[262] The spiritual formation that touches all aspects of the human person in the provider equips them to help "breathe new life" into their patients and allows the practitioner to be renewed.

Until now, spirituality has been defined too narrowly, in my perspective. It has been described as the dry bones without understanding the dynamism and the process of self-reflection, self-awareness, group support, and mentoring that bring spirituality and spiritual care to life in clinical practice. In many ways, as certain healthcare disciplines have sought to include spiritual aspects of life into their respective assessments, they have struggled to define it,[263] disagreed in knowing how to assess for it in the life contexts of patients, and how to support professional development to offer spiritual care.[264]

The process of training professionals to provide spiritual care begins with the understanding that health and human formation must encompass the biopsychosocial and spiritual aspects of individuals. Developing the ability to address spirituality requires practitioners to grow in all four dimensions of a human being over time with reflection and support, according to the USCCB.[265] What follows is a proposed formation schema for dietitians and lifestyle medicine professionals that involves developing skills of individual self-reflection on personal reactions and the provision of care, greater self-awareness, and objective savvy from participating in group support and mentoring from professionals who also practice spiritual care. Growth happens from knowing more, from seeing them practiced, and from reflecting and implementing the insights that follow. The competencies are learned, integrated into practice, and, once cultivated into a personal style, get applied creatively to a widening circle of people based on our role. Practitioners mature in living out and growing their spiritual capacity.

In many ways, the capacity described in sacred texts illustrates how the transcendent force or spirit unifies the body systems, aligning them in harmony with new energy. Ideally, well-being means that the body systems function in balance with human motivation. Health is three-dimensional: it encompasses the body, the psyche, and the social abilities shaped by spirituality, as the whole is greater than the sum of its parts

# CHAPTER 12

*The First Step to Learning the Process*

*of Working Spiritually*

## How practitioners mature in professional identity and engage in spiritual conversation

The emphasis now is on moving from definitions to describing and initiating the process of personal growth that enables dietitians and healthcare providers to provide holistic care to patients from diverse faith backgrounds. This requires a renewed understanding of the journey of developing a professional identity as a practitioner throughout one's career. More than just recognizing that spiritual needs exist and that positive spirituality influences health positively, clinicians must engage in ongoing personal growth and clinical formation to provide effective spiritual care. Nursing literature shows the negative consequences nurses often face after participating in a one-time assignment or training session on spiritual care, which leads to challenges in meeting spiritual needs.[266] Clinical formation goes beyond cognitive understanding; it involves developing the clinician's personal qualities and character, which directly affects the care they provide.

Practitioners need to receive support, mentoring, and clinical formation in the action of patient care, which helps them grow in cultural competency, morals, attentiveness to themselves, the needs of patients, critical curiosity, and adaptive flexibility.[267] The dedication of dietitians and other healthcare providers goes "beyond a job and is rooted in altruism."[268] Personal development, particularly spiritual growth, is integral to both professional advancement and a sense of calling. Dietitians undermine their own potential without realizing they are "defined not only by what they must know and do, but most importantly by a profound sense of what the physician (or dietitian) must be."[269] Robert Popovich, an accomplished clinical supervisor in Clinical Pastoral Education, said it best: "Spiritual care is an integrative corollary to being a Registered Dietitian."[270]

The growth in professional identity occurs after providers develop "reflective habits of mind, heart, and practice."[271] This enables them to understand the role of spirituality and coping in life, as well as their own needs, wounds, and emotions, which can be triggered while providing care. Inviting patients into deeper conversations—not as trauma therapists or counselors, but as supportive, knowledgeable companions and clinicians—affects patients' adjustment to illness and enhances their physical, emotional, and social well-being. Once practitioners learn to embody and live the fruits of their self-reflection and self-awareness, they can cultivate a sense of "practical wisdom" that translates "theory into an internalized identity"[272] as someone who forms "healing relationships" with the patients they serve.[273]

This practical wisdom that stems from internalizing this sense of inner coherence promotes an ability to form an "active personal presence," a term described by Dr. Gordon Hilsman.[274] Active personal presence is the radical emotional availability to patients and the wisdom that follows that allows clinicians to recognize the personal and spiritual needs of their patients and draw them to more readily share feelings, struggles, hesitations, and needs that dwell under the surface. These unaddressed issues can impact health, well-being, and motivation to implement healthy habits. As was examined earlier, unresolved grief, spiritual distress, or even the unexamined life can cause upheaval and health challenges in patients' lives as well as in practitioners.' The unexamined life with its upsets, victories, traumas, rejections, and strengths can be the "source of many hindrances in our caregiving relationships"[275] and can "lead to distress, disengagement, depression and burnout for physicians (health care providers)."[276] This can happen even if caregivers are spiritual or religious. When practitioners refresh their own awareness of their own vulnerability and personal issues, they become equipped to help others in this way.

Active presence goes beyond engaged listening. When practitioners are fully present with their clients, they not only listen and offer empathetic reflections but also invite the patient to explore their authentic selves and address what troubles them. These empathetic caregivers understand when to gently confront and draw upon their clinical knowledge, behavioral science, and spiritual perspectives. This combined empathy and wisdom foster an environment of openness for the client. Clinicians develop this capacity by processing their own lives and experiences outside of patient care, ensuring that their needs, wounds, or biases do not cloud their perceptions and assessments during patient interactions. "Through conversation and reflection, they more readily can appraise a person's strengths, needs, and ways of maintaining their own human spirits."[277]

Practicing spiritual care within a healthcare discipline is not simply about adhering to a conversational protocol for spiritual discussions. Each provider approaches this differently. Rather, it focuses on developing a professional identity and the ability to provide sensitive, profoundly reflective care. Spirituality is mainly recognized through feelings and their underlying concerns, values, attitudes, and habitual assumptions. It stems from perceptions and the essence of the experience.[278] Spiritual caregiving begins with building rapport, which goes beyond casual conversation; however, this verbal exchange can quickly address core issues since time is crucial in clinical care.

## The basics of a spiritually oriented conversation

Many of us know the importance of building rapport with our clients so they feel comfortable in telling us what we need to know about them to provide medical care. As has been described before, this is more diagnostic listening, listening in order to diagnose and provide medical care. What we are discussing here is the process of having a spiritually oriented conversation, a conversation that can provide that deeper level of healing in the patient beneath the medications, the nutrients, and the inflammation. While we use many of the same skills, empathy, questions, and supportive presence, we want to intentionally tweak these attributes of patient care in such a way that patients come to deeper insights themselves about what matters most to them.

In a later section, we will examine ways we might unknowingly side-track this from taking place in our rather unconscious reactions, here, we want to describe and illustrate what sets a spiritual conversation apart from social chatter or medically oriented discourse. While in diagnostic listening, practitioners ask questions to gather data, in spiritual care listening, this does not disappear, it is used much less often. A key to spiritually oriented healing conversation is learn to focus on the emotions and needs of the person in front of you, to listen with your heart exposed so you can communicate to them that you are aware of what they are experiencing. Consider your own reaction to their situation, and allow yourself to be moved by their plight as someone coming alongside them or as a companion on the journey. This helps you build rapport with them and extend yourself in altruism.

Caregivers may open the spiritual conversation with a question, "What's that like for you? What sense do you make of this? What recharges and motivates you?" This is followed by listening, maybe reflecting what you hear back to them or clarifying what they shared. Caregivers are attempting to zero in on the emotions that the client shares. As was stated before, spirituality is often recognized by the emotions that surface: fear, doubt, joy, hope, peace. Listen for this and learn to pause.

This lingering, or the 5–8 second pause is a central aspect of spiritual conversation.

We are attempting to open the door for them to go deeper beneath the surface where life energies can experience healing. As Hilsman states, we want "to give the patient time to consider what to share next, and almost invariably leads to the deepening of the conversation." Empathetic responses from the provider can encourage what is "happening inside the patient to further come forth."[279]

Sometimes, when a practitioner is attempting something new, and they are nervous, they ask too many questions, engage in hyperverbal sharing or focus on themselves too much. All want to be avoided as they sidetrack the client's deeper reflection. Too many questions give the provider control of the interaction but often narrow or cut the conversation short. Spiritual conversations are not social chit-chat but conversations focused on the patient and their deeper reactions and needs.

Furthermore, dietitians and providers want to remain alert to subtle communication patterns where they may project an air of superiority or moralism. With experience with this spiritually focused interchange can balance emotional involvement which portrays empathy with boundaries that prevent over-involvement with the client. Hilsman calls this functioning "in the zone of helpfulness." These conversations don't have to take a lot of time once the provider knows how to dance into this zone with a simple curiosity or question, linger, pause, reflect, share information requested by the patient, or provide clarification. Interestingly, because the provider has the medical knowledge, spiritual care can often reduce the patient's anxiety in addition to helping them get in touch with what's really bothering them as the provider can eventually provide helpful perspectives. Because stressed people often oscillate between minimization and over-exaggeration of their situation, they often benefit from compassionate normalizing feedback or information that can provide "realistic perspectives when the situation is rather common so patients don't have to feel embarrassed or worried."[280]

Developing the art of care comes from a training model called clinical formation, which is derived from Clinical Pastoral Education. Hillsman describes this learning method as one that emphasizes experience over thought, emotion over patterned behavior, and process over discussion. For the past 100 years, Clinical Pastoral Education has trained Board Certified Healthcare Chaplains to serve within healthcare systems, assisting those who are suffering or undergoing significant changes.

We apply this model to the professional development of dietitians, nutritionists, and other healthcare providers. This novel suggestion proposes that training can be offered to Registered Dietitians, Nutritionists, and other healthcare practitioners, equipping them to provide spiritual care within their specific scopes and understand when to refer a client to a Healthcare Chaplain. While this application is not entirely new, it has been implemented at Harvard Medical School, where fourth-year medical students were paired with CPE divinity students for four weeks. This collaboration aimed to impart CPE principles and emphasize the importance for medical students to critically examine their religious and spiritual convictions, as well as to explore self-awareness through writing spiritual autobiographies and reflection papers about their motivations and values.[281]

Additionally, an interesting study in Denmark exposed a cohort of hospice nurses to a process of observation in practice, reflection on praxis, action in praxis, and evaluation of action.[282] This experience taught the nurses that trusting their relational skills could enhance spiritual care. In this context, practitioners across various fields recognize that their primary tools for care and life are their own personalities, life experiences, and culture, once reflected upon, alongside their clinical knowledge

## Personal, Spiritual Timeline

To start this process, you can return to and gather your reflections on transcendence from Chapter 1, on what resonated with you on spirituality in Chapter 2, and on spiritual distress and aspects on grief that you came to notice from the discussion in Chapter 6. Use these insights and reflections and add more to make a timeline of the events of your life by decades. Use the sample timeline at the end of this chapter to collect the events of your life and spiritual journey. Think about your experiences and your encounter with the divine, or the high points of your experiences and the difficult times. Add in the emotions you may have remembered feeling and about what happened in the events or experiences. Don't discount anything as insignificant; as you reflect, record what surfaces in your memory and heart. Above this line, make a parallel timeline where you remember any spiritual or religious experiences you may have had, even starting in early childhood. One early memory I recorded on my timeline was my memory of awakening early every morning before anyone else. I tiptoed quietly, sat behind a poofy chair, so no one could see me, and gazed for about 15 minutes out the picture window of my parent's living room. It overlooked some beautiful grass-covered hills with a brick house at the top of the hill in the distance, like a Grant Wood painting. At that time, I thought about things and felt centered, safe, in awe of the great expanse before me, and close to God. This memory tempered what came next from the same time period, the memory of my grandmother, who had moved in with us, as she was dying of cancer, being rushed to the hospital in the middle of the night due to low potassium. All the adults, my parents, aunts, and uncles who were visiting, were crying, hugging each other, and ignoring the kids. In this memory, I felt insignificant, anxious, fearful, and really sad. Grandma's bedroom was right next to mine, and I had just watched a TV show with her a few hours before. I learned that beauty surrounded me, but I had to deal with my own emotions because no one noticed. These thoughts made me strive to be heard. They came forward during my experience of Clinical Pastoral Education and motivated me as a chaplain to obtain advanced certification as a grief specialist.

This learning process, according to Hilsman, helps caregivers become familiar with their own troubling and triumphant stories, preparing them to better hear the stories of others. Throughout the writing of their timeline, Hilsman encourages caregivers to look for three kinds of narratives from their lives to remember and reflect on: their heritage stories, which incorporate early influences from the natural world, parents, teachers, relatives, pastors, and authorities; the stories shaped by their developing values, beliefs, decisions, and commitments from their growing cognitions, pondering, study, and discourse; and stories from remarkable encounters, referring to experiences of transcendence that may have caused them feelings of ecstasy or misery. Heritage stories generally set the stage for what people seek and value later in life. Much of what hinders a person's caregiving relationships and capacity for intimacy comes from unresolved early thoughts and values.[283]

As you create your timeline and reflect on various events, experiences, thoughts, feelings, and spiritual encounters, you may begin to notice recurring feelings, ways your spirit has been supported, or how you have carried burdens related to these events over the years. For instance, consider a dietitian with unresolved grief and buried painful childhood memories of their grandmother, like mine, who works in an oncology unit. They might unintentionally project their discomfort with loss onto their patients, avoiding discussions about death and associated feelings. Alternatively, they could experience emotional transference, feeling deeply moved by an older woman who reminds them of their grandmother. The purpose of this timeline is to help you understand your emotional reactions, coping patterns, and how your personal history influences your current relationships.[284]

Caregivers also tend to relate to patients in the same way they relate to themselves.[285] For example, someone who often intellectualizes their own feelings may minimize the time they allow a patient to talk about their feelings and instead offer suggestions to divert attention away from them by providing information.

## The importance of clarifying your own spiritual perspectives

If the goal of the interaction is spiritual care, the provider needs to clarify their own convictions and philosophy regarding spirituality and religion. Without this clarity, they may not be able to facilitate spiritual care effectively. Many providers feel that their spiritual perspectives are insufficient to care for others, which can reflect a helpful humility and a desire for growth. As Popovich states, "This is the time that we want to admit our ignorance."[286] Keep in mind from the earlier discussion, spirituality looks at the core ways a person gathers their life essence, experiences, feelings and purpose together to find meaning, contribution, delight in living and relationship with the transcendence or God. It has also been said that to help a grieving or distressed person, the empathetic individual must "enter the wilderness of their experience with them."[287] How effective can this care be if the provider lacks their own guidance or "compass" as they listen and support the patient in what troubles them? Providers recognize clients' spiritual questions after addressing their own earlier dilemmas, and often clinicians can discern the first steps for clients to take.

Using the previous examples of spiritual conversations in nutrition counseling, as shown in the sample verbatims, notice what I highlighted as spiritual issues that surfaced. I spoke about listening for clues to what matters most to the client, their sense of meaning, purpose, connection to the divine. The first portion of the book includes several written spiritual assessment instruments that you can become familiar with. By exploring different spiritual assessment tools, you'll become able to formulate your own spiritual listening frame developed by working with your own life narrative and those of your clients. This frame will help you to notice the heart of the spiritual matter at hand. Developing or rejuvenating an early framework is a means for understanding people. Reviewing the information on the basic tenets of the world religions will also help expand your spiritual frame of reference to adapt to those outside of your personal experiences.

I remember working with a man from Tibet at an addiction center who was Hindu. He shared how he calmed himself by quieting his mind and praying with his japa mala beads. I included this in his lifestyle plan to help him manage stress. He was very devout and clearly wanted to connect his faith to his life goals. This suggestion came from listening to him rather than recommending another evidence-based practice.

If providers are emotionally available and spiritually alert, spiritual insights for the patient often arise within them as they listen to clients. An image, Scripture, or song may come to mind. How often has this occurred in my own care encounters? For example, as a client spoke, I kept thinking of the words from the 23rd Psalm. I said, "The words 'The Lord is my shepherd' keep coming to my mind." The client burst into tears and said, "My grandmother always read that to me when I was falling asleep. She is with me right now!" For another client, a beautiful mountainside kept filling my mind; when I shared that, the client beamed and said, "That is where I always find peace! I'm going to remember my last time hiking. That will comfort me."

For another client, who I mentioned earlier, as part of lifestyle medicine, I invited a Native American Medicine Man to the long-term care room to burn sacred sage before continuing our discussion on healthy eating. This connected the patient to what mattered most to him—his connection to the Great Spirit—and motivated him to try new foods because it was important to him now.

As you reflect on this, challenge yourself to create a plan to regularly nurture your receptivity or spiritual openness. Use some of the supplemental spiritual activities, such as poetry, meditations, sacred Scripture, or worship from your own background. A common approach is to read the text three times: the first time, simply note what the text conveys; the second time, pay attention to what stands out and resonates with you; and the third time, consider what inspires you to take action in your life. This process is known as sacred reading, but it can also be practiced with a piece of music or while viewing a work of art.

If you do not have a religious or spiritual background to return to, pay attention to those around you—at work or in your activities—who have touched you with their kindness. Ask them what they do for spiritual growth and consider joining them. Alternatively, experiment with different faith traditions to see how they resonate with you. You could also make an effort to spend time in nature regularly and observe how it nurtures your spirit. Read classical poetry or sacred writings and notice what inspires you. My only caution is that, from my perspective, humans may experience fragmentation if the goal is merely to seek nothingness. Always aim to find peace, care, and something more within your experience that comes from the positive force in living. For me, I refer to that place as God. For some, it exists within themselves;

for others, it's the transcendent force that accompanies and inspires them. A positive spiritual presence, God, integrates and inspires. It does not bring fear, fragmentation, or grandiosity from this author's experience of spiritual care and direction.

Sometimes, as adults, we can revisit our roots and take a fresh look to see where to start. In seeking independence, some may hastily discard important parts of their religious heritage. A thoughtful reconsideration of an earlier faith can be much less anxiety-inducing than adopting something entirely different from what we have known. I remember an Iowa farmer who raised pigs and was Lutheran. He was spiritually befuddled after working previously with a dietitian via Telehealth who had suggested that he try transcendental meditation and Ayurveda-style vegetarian eating. He could not figure out what to do. Were these suggestions serving him or the provider from Chicago whom he had spoken with? When dietitians bring up ways spiritual needs can be met, they need to listen for clues from the patients themselves for what they suggest. It seems possible that the dietitian was projecting what helped her or someone else with vastly different needs and experiences. The goal, from my experience, is not to wow the person with the most novel practice but to listen for what you see in the flow of the other's life and experience when you suggest a spiritual practice for rebalancing life.

I often hear dietitians identify as faith-based and state that they pray with most patients because it is what the patients desire. While I support prayer, it is not always the first step in addressing spiritual needs. As Hilsman notes, "Not everyone wants prayer or needs it," and automatic praying can feel "more like taking refuge in a comfortable action for the caregiver than meeting the patient in her current difficult uniqueness."[288] Before a provider prays with a patient, it may be best for the caregiver to take a few seconds to center themselves, as long as the patient has not requested prayer. This brief moment of reflection allows the caregiver to listen more attentively and offer a prayer that resonates with what they have heard from the patient. This approach requires flexibility and a provider's ability to access their own depth and spirituality to ensure the prayer is genuinely beneficial for the client. Additionally, it may necessitate that dietitians or any providers release the need to control or strictly adhere to a certain way of doing things.

The goals of these early experiences, including the timeline and spiritual growth and reflection activities, are to enhance your sensitivity and self-awareness. Ideally, this journey is not undertaken alone; it connects you with a supportive small group of trusted peers and a facilitator who can help you understand yourself and the impact of your interactions with others. A model of this will be shared in the next chapter, along with the supportive experience and training offered by The Renewed Practitioner Training. This small group differs from individual or group therapy and is distinct from typical clinical supervision, as it includes theological and spiritual reflection, making it more than just a clinical support group.

You can form a group of trusted peers who are equally ready to grow in self-awareness regarding their lives and healthcare practices. Take turns facilitating the group discussions and sharing your clinical examples, giving each person a chance to present and facilitate. If someone expresses strong emotion, acknowledge their feelings process the experience together or consider discussing it with a counselor to continue your healing process.

A common thought right here is that the process is like having psychotherapy in a group in the midst of clinical formation. This is not exactly correct. The focus of clinical formation and this timeline and later, the verbatim conversations with clients presented to the group, is not like psychotherapy in focusing on healing the clinician themselves but on assessing the quality of the clinical encounter to heal the client.[289]

# Personal Timeline

- On the timeline below, reflect on major life experiences, both positive and negative, by decade. Mark and label the timeline for these experiences on the bottom line.

- On the top line, do the same for important spiritual experiences by decade. This may be experiences of deep peace, community connection, or relationship with the divine, nature or positive force in living.

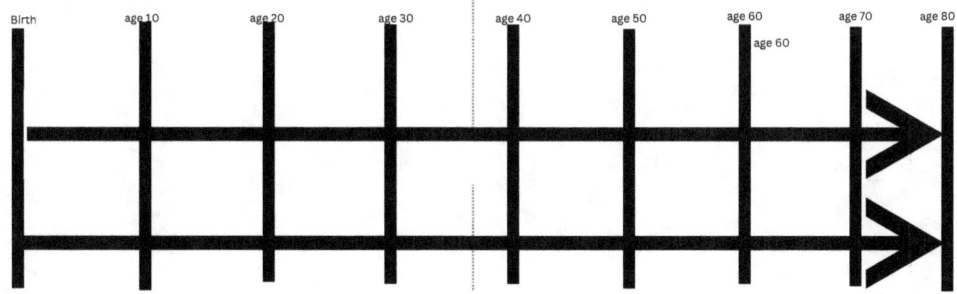

# CHAPTER 13

*The Core of Clinical Process Learning:*

*Reflecting on the Clinical Encounter*

A key step in clinical formation, as described by Hilsman, is capturing your interaction with a client in written form, as closely as possible to what actually took place, and bringing it to your small group for processing. (We will describe the parameters for this small group in the next section.) This approach demonstrates how the "real patient care experience is used to educate."[290] Early in the development of methods in Clinical Pastoral Education (CPE), the focus shifted from examining case studies to writing verbatims, as this was more effective for learning and growth from clinical encounters. Verbatims are typically written documents; however, some are experimenting with virtual seminars in place of this intensive writing process to facilitate learning. The goal is not for the group to grade your performance but to engage with you in this recaptured clinical encounter so you can learn. This process helps you understand how your reactions, responses, attitudes, and biases—even if unvoiced—impacted your interaction with the client.

This process enables you to develop a "renewed professional caregiving style beyond social diagnostics or merely tolerant interaction" and helps you assess whether you operated in a "zone of helpfulness or were under or over-involved" with the client at that moment.[291] Presenting a verbatim account, processing it with peers, and reflecting on it can truly enhance your maturity in caregiving and clarify what was achieved during the session. Haven't you always wondered how things went, especially with those clients who challenged you?

These situations—those with emotional complexity or uncertainty, or moments when you felt truly amazed by the outcome—are very beneficial to discuss in a group setting. These written accounts facilitate active learning for both the presenter and the group members, who will critique and engage with the presenter during the discussion. Hilsman notes, "CPE uses the context of human difficulties so participants can recognize the radical challenges." These radical challenges shine a light on areas within you, the provider, where you experience pain, underdevelopment, narrow perspectives, or strengths. The goal is to develop "an emotional awareness of interpersonal dynamics" between you and others, as this allows access to "other people's depths," where genuine healing and motivation occur. When dietitians actively encourage personal sharing from their clients, they tap into a positive and motivating resource rather than remaining stuck and blaming the patient for having low readiness to change. These types of encounters build trust in patients and help them feel known as a person.

The process goes as follows: first, you write up an appropriate situation in a verbatim, and reflect upon it to notice what comes forth for you; second, you present it to the group and hear their reactions, thoughts, challenges, validations, and questions that send you to a quiet corner to reflect again, to consider how to address the issue and craft some pointed goals for your next interactions. In essence, we use our weaknesses to grow and our honest reflections to be validated. Peers draw attention to incongruencies that can keep our interchanges with patients "chatty, confusing, superficial or grandiosely over instructive."[292] If we are truthful, is that not a reason dietitians so often default back to an instructional mode? They may not know how to linger or why to invite clients to address anything deeper, maybe because they have not explored these issues in themselves.

Some aspects to consider alone after writing a verbatim but before you present to the small group of peers:[293]

- Was what I said and what I did congruent?
- Do I notice a pattern that keeps the relationship superficial
- What did I like about the interaction? What did I say or do?
  What would I do differently?
- What did the person need emotionally and spiritually from me? Are they
  spiritually distressed or grieving? How do they recharge themselves or do they?
- Who would be best to provide it?
- What sacred/poetic writings come to mind about this conversation?
- Are there any cultural implications that will impact my supportive nutritional
  care of this patient?

Determine where you would appreciate the small group exploring with you and list that as a focus point. Notice yourself: Do you tend to have empathetic interactions, or do you tend to move to the intellectual plane more quickly than necessary?

Rather than a scorecard, these reflection questions are meant to help you become aware of yourself as a caregiver and understand how your own attitudes, values, assumptions, strengths, and weaknesses impact your emotional and active presence with clients. A key skill in maturing in professional competency to offer spiritual care as well as clinical care is learning how to function as a member of a group of colleagues and how to seek consultation with peers. The hope from this structured process of self-reflection and interactive processing is that you become more able to work with conflict constructively and understand the broader picture of what is impacting your client's health, nutrition and self-care needs. This broader understanding can include developing a greater appreciation of the client's social conditions and social determinants of health.

Clinical formation using a verbatim is a key aspect of breathing life into the learning process for healthcare providers to offer spiritual care and engage with clients around their spirituality in the pursuit of wellness. Individual reflection, followed by group processing and support, and personal reflection are key aspects of the "observation, reflection, action, and evaluation of action" method described with the Danish hospice nurses and the methodology described in this work, which is acclimated from Clinical Pastoral Education.

This learning is best done in a small group with a trained facilitator who is also working outside of the group with their own supervision. For example, in The Renewed Practitioner Spiritual Care training process, each participant will take on the roles of both presenter and group member and be guided by a trained facilitator. To get started, as described earlier, consider gathering a small group of other healthcare professionals who desire to develop their personal capacities to practice emotively and engage with the client's deeper needs or spiritual needs and take turns presenting verbatims, serving as group members and facilitators. Assure everyone that the space is confidential and a means to develop oneself as a provider of healthcare that promotes whole-person healing. This format can assist clinicians to grow in personal insight, spiritual maturity and ability to promote real healing in their clients.

# CHAPTER 14

*The Power of Peer-Group Learning*

*for the Lifestyle Medicine Practitioner*

## How the small group members assist your learning

Peer group learning is a key ingredient that has been missing from spiritual care training. This is the model of CPE, where personal reflections from life and later from clinical encounters will be explored to understand the feelings and behaviors of caring that result. In this way, peers do not discuss the interaction with you or the timeline of the clinical encounter. Instead, they process these experiences with you, offering honest thoughts, reactions, critiques, and sometimes validation. They may place themselves in your position regarding the timeline or the client during the verbatim presentation. This helps them recognize the impact of your verbal and non-verbal responses, allowing you to learn from your interactions. Although dietitians are part of a profession that promotes wellness and spiritual vitality, providers best learn the skills of delivering spiritual care by examining and engaging with interactions that demand more from them: in a "context of human difficulties...to consider changes that may need to be made."[294]

By following the flow of the stories, group members assist the presenter in recognizing where the flow changed unnecessarily or unintentionally, and where they moved away from the particulars of the spiritual conversation. Later, reflecting on the feedback may help you understand what in yourself and your story caused this shift. Certain group rules, agreed upon before the group starts, help ensure that the group is most supportive to both the presenter and the participants. This group process is not intended to hurt anyone; however, it must allow members to provide honest feedback about what they perceived or observed during the session. The goal is for each participant to grow and eliminate communication patterns that impede effective patient care. The notion of being a nice, compliant group member to maintain harmony should be discarded and replaced with a commitment to authenticity and honest, specific questioning and observations in feedback and critique. This means that conflict among group members will be a part of the learning process.

Learning how to negotiate conflict and, at times, engage in it becomes a very useful skill in a dietitian's or lifestyle medicine provider's personal life and professional career. Healthcare can be a conflict-rich environment, depending on where it is and the formation of the other team members. Patient needs, stress, and expectations of other providers can often be high.

Some providers may exhibit inflated egos and symptoms of what Balboni calls the hidden agenda. He defines the hidden agenda as a culture of privilege arising from misguided socialization that some team members experience, often exacerbated by burnout. This results in "poor behavior that devalues and objectifies patients and rigid hierarchical relationships that limit correction of abuses of power."[295] Learning to assess one's own skills and vulnerabilities can help dietitians and healthcare providers become more resilient and open to healthy human interactions. (Consider the benefits of clinical formation, especially in light of the low professional morale previously noted among some dietitians and medical providers in general.)

Personal reflection, small group sharing, and feedback are not therapy, just as spiritual care is not therapy but rather a supportive presence that helps clients overcome barriers to self-discovery and realizing their potential. Groups serve as a vital support system and a place for learning. They allow old behaviors to be observed, new behaviors to be attempted, and opportunities to learn from peers and supervisors to be directly experienced and integrated.[296] Small group processing assists providers in integrating spiritual care into their practice and helps them connect their lives and identities into a cohesive whole to find greater meaning. It also enables them to set focused goals to address their typical challenges and strengthen their existing skills.

### What role does the group facilitator play in processing the verbatim?

The role of the peer group facilitator is to keep the peer group focused on processing the clinical encounter. This is not a group discussion of the clinical encounter presented in the verbatim, a social conversation or group therapy, just like a spiritual conversation is not therapy, although when a group member gets the opportunity to facilitate the group they may watch for some similar dynamics.

Just like any of the group members, the facilitator wants to put themselves into the role of the client to notice the back-and-forth movements of the interchange and how that impacts them. They want to notice if the professional asks many questions, shares unduly about their own situation, seems to remain shallow in their engagement with the client, or swings into over-involvement, which may portray loose boundaries.

As summarized from Hilsman, 2018, the facilitator, along with the other peer group members, also needs to notice any unexpected and rather unconscious interplay in the session's dynamics. Does the presenter seem overly identified with the patient? This could make them unable to assess the patient's situation realistically. Does the presenter describe the client unduly positively, or negatively? Does the client seem excessively connected or averse to the provider, which may signal transference? And, is the presenter themselves, distorted in their reaction towards the client, ascribing strongly worded attributions that do not seem warranted to the objective listening? This could signal countertransference. And, lastly, do you sense that the presenter is projecting their own situation onto the client?

Recall the example from this author's explanation of the timeline exercise and her own painful experience with the death of her grandmother. If this provider had not processed her own feelings of loss and grief, she could have overreacted emotionally to an older woman client with cancer who came to her in the clinic.

As the peer group facilitator, you also have a responsibility that you share with the other peer group members to care for the presenter to facilitate the group as a safe place to share. How will you offer critique to colleagues that supports their growth while at the same time does not wound or discourage them? This can be brought out and described in group norms at the start of the group. Your role will be to notice if the group is veering away from this.

The process of writing and sharing an account of a patient encounter can make a provider feel very vulnerable. We should not be ashamed of our ignorance or our weaknesses and struggles. Many providers are accustomed to the patterns and personal styles they have developed from caring for patients over the years. Hilsman describes that opening up "can be very jarring," but it is an act of courage with a purpose: to leave behind old ways of relating and to see oneself anew, both professionally and personally. It is quite normal to feel defensive but allow yourself to be impacted by the group experience. Avoid the temptation that science-based healthcare providers often face to return to the cognitive realm, where you feel more comfortable. You will learn by confronting what lies within you, allowing for a less encumbered relationship with clients. There is real growth that comes from "honestly standing face to face" with the probing questions posed by group members, who will also validate certain aspects of you as they become aware of them.

Group members will support you when feelings arise during the sharing of personal dimensions of your professional and personal life function.

As you engage in the process of closely examining your life story and spiritual experiences, it is most effective in a safe group with a trusted facilitator. Each participant is assisted in integrating their feelings and experiences, which fosters greater self-awareness and spiritual growth. Hilsman describes this as the "goal of sharing our stories in clinical learning encounters, which can be seen as guiding us towards integration." This understanding helps us comprehend ourselves better and clarifies what our clients are trying to achieve when facing a health issue or attempting to change their daily habits for better health.

What are you trying to integrate into your life in order to animate your practice with spiritual care? You may be carrying "uneven scattered shards of religious or spiritual teaching, practices or beliefs, a history of past efforts of helping people in discomfort, some awareness of psychological issues or therapeutic modes, along with values, biases, attitudes, assumptions and patterns of communication"[297] More than likely, you have not learned how to hold these together in a working therapeutic manner.

You may find that what you offer to most of your patients is helpful, yet you might not feel effective in helping them achieve their goals. Reflect on the mind/body practices you have suggested. Are these recommendations based on what the patient has shared with you, or do you consistently suggest yoga or slow-breathing mindfulness practices simply because you've read about their benefits? We should be cautious of providers who have "one pill for every illness."[298]

You may be getting signs that you need to explore some imbalances inside of you: you feel confident that you are offering evidence-based proficient care but notice frequent no-shows or that your patients seem to routinely be faltering in making lasting lifestyle changes. This significant discrepancy was noted in a moderate-size study (n=133 patients, n=180 dietitians) which rated dietitians for depth of relationship, shared decision-making, and facility for offering holistic care.[299] Dietitians rated themselves much higher than patients did in terms of communication, holistic approaches, and personalized care, as well as in their understanding of patients. Lacking the skills to recognize their own vulnerabilities or weaknesses, dietitians believed they were performing better than they truly were.

Rather than a process of focusing on evidence-based care and improving the concrete health markers alone, this experience of clinical process formation allows providers to bring along the human elements and include spiritual care beneath the science. This effective and efficacious paradigm of caring for the whole person allows the provider to become "a skilled caregiver who is learning the art of informally helping people overcome the barriers to telling of the as yet untold stories" that impact their care and follow-through with health-enhancing behaviors.[300]

## How you learn being a small group member

As you participate as a member of a small group, you venture to gain new skills and clinical awareness by exploring your peer's clinical encounters. A good way to zero in on the ebb and flow of the encounter can be to label the types of responses your peer is using to address the patient: did they ask a question, provide support, reflect or provide information. While patients come to providers to learn new information and behaviors, research has shown, summarized earlier, that they also come for emotional support and to find new perspectives for bringing life together with health.

Empathetic care may start with a question like, "How are you dealing with this?" But truly supportive providers listen more than they speak. Moments of pause or as Hilsman describes, "professional lingering" during patients' intimate sharing invites them to go deeper, to get to what is the linchpin of their difficulties.[301]

Hilsman describes this *lingering* that dietitians can benefit from as a few seconds of quiet after a patient's disclosure or a piece of education that allows a patient to "deepen their disclosure."[302] In social conversation, it can become customary to fill in the moments of silence which "truncates because time is of the essence or the person is considering what they will say next, or to offer their own point of view or to follow the counseling protocol of a clarifying response." This "interpersonal waiting" is strategically situated and demonstrates attention and genuine care. Ask yourself, are you "professionally and interpersonally curious" or do you too quickly default to information giving?

As you listen to a colleague's verbatim conversation, what do you notice in the flow of back-and-forth responses? Does the dietitian ask many questions and allow pauses for patient contemplation, feelings, and consideration? Or do they tend to give information before fully exploring the patient's experience? Did the patient continue to share on a deeper, more intimate level, or did they remain focused on surface issues? Was the clinician able to invite the client to discuss their experiences and feelings, including what discourages them? Is grief or spiritual distress being expressed, or are they maintaining a stiff upper lip while coping with food in a dysfunctional way? Look for patterns where the provider may steer the conversation back to topics they are more comfortable with. Do they revert to being the expert, or do they connect with the patient through shared human experiences that show personal care? Also, reflect on whether you exhibit any of these less-than-optimal patterns in your own interactions with your patients?

Share your reflections and observations with the presenter, including the questions that developed inside you and the emotions that surfaced as you listened. Also, share your observations of any patterns you saw. For example, maybe every time the patient voiced an emotion, the provider spoke or asked a question. Are you afraid of creating conflict with the presenter or offending her? This helps you consider your own tolerance of and approach to conflict. This is not a time for flattery, but honest validation is also helpful if you see a helpful response and pattern.

After the group meeting, both the presenter and group members can benefit from taking a few moments to reflect and recharge. Going for a short walk or spending some quiet time alone can be quite helpful. Consider the emotional moments of the group: what words stood out, and how do you feel about the person who expressed them? What issues were addressed, and what did you notice within yourself? This type of small group interaction focuses on the presenter, their personalities, history, feelings, and needs, and how these elements impacted the clinical interaction. If conflicts arose, they can be addressed and processed during another small group meeting interaction.

This type of learning is self-directed, personal, and requires readiness to be vulnerable and authentic. The formation exercises described so far necessitate robust honesty with oneself and the ability to reflect on your experiences, values, and faith perspectives. This self-reflection leads to greater self-awareness. Additionally, it is essential to cultivate certain desires: inviting oneself to tolerate conflict and caring enough to offer pointed observations and feelings to others, addressing their needs and issues as they arise. This learning occurs at the right time and place.

Furthermore, developing your own sense of spirituality or alignment with a religious perspective enables you to recognize and engage more effectively with the spiritual concerns of others who may have different beliefs. This doesn't mean you have to adopt a religious viewpoint if you feel differently; however, being open to considering the spiritual dimensions of life—such as in nature, the arts, music, interpersonal relationships, and within yourself—can be very beneficial and a good place to start.

These capacities allow you to develop certain clinical skills that facilitate offering spiritual care within nutrition or other healthcare discipline. These skills may not have been part of a provider's initial professional formation, which may have focused on evidence-based clinical skill-based care, nutrition education, or how to offer support in general or with motivational interviewing. Clinical care for most disciplines has addressed the biopsychosocial aspects of treatment, leaving off spirituality. Spirituality facilitates forming a life coherence, binding diverse aspects of care together in a working whole.

Another important skill that surfaces in clinical process formation is for the provider to develop the capacity to grieve and welcome mourning in their clients. Remember that Wolfelt described working with carried grief "like going into the wilderness." If a provider has not worked toward healing their own life losses, they will be hampered and not be available to welcome this in their clients.[303] Using this reference and the support of a clinical learning small group can provide some context that supports some catch-up grieving. If a provider notices in themselves a pattern of repressed grief or unfinished grieving, it may help them be more clinically and emotionally available to their patients if they get support through counseling and some prescribed time for their own self-reflection. Professionals often need to linger in their own wilderness to heal.

Many clinicians listen to patients mainly to gather relevant details for care, rather than taking an overview of the client's life. This approach can cause them to overlook important human elements that contribute to health, well-being, and flourishing. The ability to build human-to-human rapport encourages you, using your personality, to intentionally develop warm, engaging relationships with a broader circle of people. When you attempt to incorporate spiritual support into nutrition counseling or another healthcare discipline, it's common to feel more comfortable offering it to those who seem familiar to you. Challenge yourself to step outside your comfort zone as you develop your approach so that everyone can benefit from holistic care. Allow moments when you're not just listening to gather information for your nutritional or physical assessment of facts and symptoms. While some information-gathering listening is necessary, if providers fail to engage in personal listening that helps patients explore what's underneath the surface, the most valuable information may go unheard. Understanding clinical processes helps you, the provider, identify where you might be less responsive to your patients.

An interesting thought about clinical process learning is that it helps awaken a new understanding and empathy for the "unique vulnerability of the patient" as well as their own "special vulnerability that comes from being one who truly gives care" as the provider.[304]

Another important aspect of active professional growth is clarifying your own religious and spiritual convictions. This was mentioned earlier in this section, but developing a sense of peace with your spirituality allows you to view health as a three-dimensional experience. Spirituality integrates the body, mind, and social skills into a cohesive whole that creates mission, meaning, purpose, and a fulfilling or flourishing life. It also highlights what may be hindered within providers and what can stimulate unhealthy habits and poor self-care in their lives as well as in their clients. (Refer to the discussion of spiritual intelligence mentioned earlier in the Preface.)

Without spiritual sensitivity or alertness, you may misunderstand your patients and think their issue is psychological when it may actually be a lack of spirituality or life coherence. Remember the Iowa farmer who was struggling to practice transcendental meditation and Ayurveda. The goal is not always to suggest something novel, but to help patients consider what works for them religiously or spiritually. To do otherwise invites greater patient anxiety. I cringe when I recall a chaplain whose goal with everyone was to "blow their minds" with something new. This emphasis often produces anxiety for many and is not the best approach in my opinion.

If you remember, the metaphor for listening for spiritual issues is like trying to recognize a cell tower along the road; some are camouflaged and resemble pine or palm trees at first glance. "Grounding your care with an assessment framework," according to Hilsman, can be very helpful. Written spiritual tools are important for providers to prepare for noticing potential spiritual issues as clients speak. You can use any of the spiritual assessment tools included in this resource. Which one you choose often depends more on your own perspectives and what you feel most comfortable listening for.

In addition to the written assessment tools, you can also refer to the list about spirituality in Chapter 3 to identify existential issues. Clients do not always need to speak about God to describe a spiritual issue that can impact their motivation and health. For some patients, I include a short list of feelings such as discouragement, fear, joy, and peace, along with a rating scale. I provide this list to clients during onboarding and when we are nearing the conclusion of addressing an issue or health concern. When clients see their scores increase for these positive attributes, most feel encouraged by the blossoming of spiritual vitality that has been developing quietly during lifestyle care. (See the Appendix for this rating scale.)

This next skill for providers of spiritual care may surprise you and leave you wondering about its relevance to lifestyle medicine. When addressing spiritual issues, developing the ability to use metaphors, sacred texts, or images can be incredibly helpful for illustrating intangible concepts to clients. These practices can significantly influence transcendental awareness and the expansion of consciousness as components of spiritual intelligence.

Remember my use of the alarm clock for life review, the cell phone tower for spiritual listening, and the sacred text from Ezekiel 37:1-10 to illustrate how spiritual care has often been viewed as a pile of bones instead of a living process of professional development. Cultivating the ability to offer spiritual care within the healthcare discipline is not just about following a recipe for making a casserole, but rather for creating a soufflé. This growth process gains momentum after receiving guidance from compassionate others and serves as a means to develop your craft or the artistic creativity and spiritual intelligence in the provision of care.

These skills help cultivate the virtues, habits of generous behavior, that allow you to offer holistic, collaborative, and empathetic care. Providers develop what Hilsman calls "an objective eye" to consider all the data from the chart, the patient, and their awareness of spirituality to interpret what they see. Metabolic syndrome may be addressed by helping the patient find deeper meaning in life as well as by additional means. This approach is much different from a dry, mechanical, evidence-based practice that lacks the warmth of human kindness or the oppressive care of an expert living with a "hidden agenda." Supercharged healthcare encourages providers to understand themselves, interpersonal dynamics, and the power of offering care that is immersive and infused with the assistance of Transcendence, a Higher Power, or, for some of us, God.

Lastly, this three-dimensional model of clinical formation has sought to animate the bones or mechanics of offering spiritual care with the power of "radical self-awareness" and encounter with transcendence, which facilitates greater emotional and spiritual maturity. Active presence comes when a person is comfortable with difficult feelings, experiences of pain, suffering, and strengths because they have encountered similar themes in their own story. Hilsman writes, "One tends to do to others' feelings what one does with one's own feelings."[305] When courage is applied to clinical care, the provider can more easily combat "emotional blindness" and bring in new light that leaves patients feeling that the provider "gets them and their situation."

This awareness operates on two levels: an immediate awareness of your own emotions in the moment and an ongoing familiarity with your life story, as it has shaped your relationships. Both dimensions of self-awareness help dietitians become more emotionally mature as they care for patients. It's helpful to remember Hilsman's suggestion: "A closer look at the relationships of all human beings would reveal the holes left in our ability to use all of our emotions fully in our relationships."[306] He notes that if a person stifles their anger, they may not notice the submerged anger affecting their patient. The goal is not emotional perfection, which is impossible, but to grow in the capacity for authenticity and altruism that helps people struggling to find greater spiritual and human vitality. Another way to describe what we seek for professionals is to say that when they engage clients, they should be "all in one place."[307]

## Additional formation experiences

When a clinician is intentional in exposing themselves to others with health issues, with higher needs or those outside of their own life experiences or culture, they can expand their current perception of reality and culture which is a strong aid to professional identity growth.[308] As has been discussed, formation in spiritual care comes from encountering differences, experiences and people and developing a deeper relationship with them, which develops both people involved. For example, in forming student nurses in Europe, Baldacchino had student nurses accompany patients who were ill on pilgrimage to Lourdes, France and the healing water and community prayer. All participants developed deeper relationships and experienced personal spiritual growth.

In this light, practitioners can stay alert to other providers who influence them with their calmness, practical wisdom, and resiliency. They should ask these providers about their lives, and shadow them, or a healthcare chaplain, to learn about their deeper motivations for practicing in healthcare and how they nurture a special presence in caring for others. Observe how spiritual conversations arise while attentively caring for the patient and the positive outcomes that result from such care. Like many spiritualities and religious traditions, growth is fueled by shared stories, experiences, and modeling spiritually impactful ways of living and practicing.

The objective of this work has been to present compelling evidence that spirituality is a positive health asset, as it impacts biology, psychology, and social functioning to motivate living life fully to flourish. We discover spirituality by removing obstacles and being courageous and attentive to encounters with transcendence and other people who move us. Spirituality comes from being touched personally and not so much from being able to define it. Practitioners become healers when they become aware of the other before them as a whole person and their care as a vehicle for growth. They also learn through self-awareness to develop skills of dealing with conflict, forming life-giving relationships with others, and personal spiritual practices themselves to replenish their own "why" for practicing.

As you explore spirituality and this clinical process formation, please keep Healthy Rise Nutrition and The Renewed Practitioner appraised of your experiences. You can contact us at mary@renewedpractitioner.com or mary@healthyrisenutrition.com.

# Group Member Reflection

**1**

### What did I learn when I put myself in the patient's place?

Did the presenter communicate with me in a way that was helpful, encouraging, shaming or unclear? Did I remember to share my honest reactions rather than discuss this from my head?

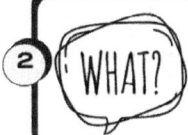

**2**

### What did I learn about spiritual care?

How did this client experience their spirituality? Did what the practitioner suggest to them (me) seem to flow and be consistent with the person? What would I suggest to this person?

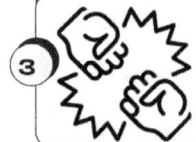

**3**

### Do I struggle to be authentic in my feedback to this peer?

Do I want to be a nice group member rather than an honest one? Do I seek harmony or to be helpful to this peer? How do I routinely handle conflict? What would I change and be intentional in future interactions.?

**4**

### Does this peer seem to welcome feedback?

I will remember that honest feedback on professional interactions can feel jarring. Does this peer welcome feedback and show a desire to grow? Do they feel egotistical?

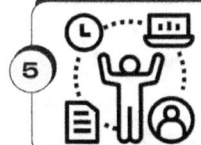

**5**

### Do I have any other insights not listed here?

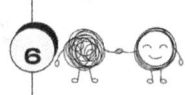

**6**

### Remember that this is not therapy!

This is not group therapy but a group of peers who desire to grow more authentic in patient and staff interactions. How can I extend myself to help my peer and myself grow?

# Group Facilitator Reflection

**1**

### How can I promote care of the presenter

While the goal of the small group is authenticity, how can I support the presenter who is making themselves vulnerable in the sharing? Are all the group members communicating respectfully but yet honestly?

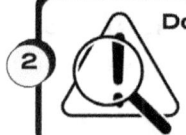

**2**

### Do I recognize any unhelpful patterns?

Does the presenter stay in a spiritually oriented interchange or do they ask questions, share excessively, divert to being the expert or share reactions to the client that are unduly positive or negative. Do they project their own experience on clients?

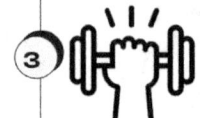

**3**

### What strengths in the presenter can I emphasize?

Do I feel warmth, empathy and would I feel open to speak to this presenter about emotionally laden topics? How did they invite the client to go deeper in sharing? Did they help the client reframe anxiety by sharing a perspective?

**4**

### Does this peer seem to welcome feedback?

I will remember that honest feedback on professional interactions can feel jarring. Does this peer welcome feedback and show a desire to grow? Do they feel egotistical?

**5**

### What did I learn about spiritual conversation from this presentation?

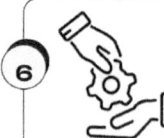

**6**

### Remember that this is not therapy!

This is not group therapy but a group of peers who desire to grow more authentic in patient and staff interactions. How can I extend myself to help my peer, the group, and myself to grow?

# APPENDIX

*Supplemental Spiritual Resources*

*for Use in Dietetic Practice*

When you consider using any supplemental spiritual practices in your nutrition counseling session, keep in mind the person's preferences in their care, and their personality factors. Do they speak easily or not about their feelings and their life experiences? Do they seem overly conscientious or compulsive in their follow-through? Are they generally agreeable to suggestions and new experiences? According to Carson et al., your awareness of their personal style needs to impact what you suggest for mind/body/spiritual practices, or the positive impact may be limited.[309] In this study, those most extroverted did better with the support that encouraged them to describe their feelings when their life experiences/narrative got to be shared in the session, while the more tight-laced, low-emotive clients relished moments of quiet mindfulness/prayer/spiritual experiences during and following the session. This insight is particularly important when the personality of practitioner and client differ.

Ask yourself, too, "What is their typical mode of engaging in life and new experiences, their typical religious or spiritual practices, level of emotional/spiritual distress? According to Carlson et al., when a person does not receive the type of supportive/spiritual care that they prefer, they may be more "disappointed and subsequently not fully [commit] themselves to the assigned intervention." "Half-hearted participation" could result in less engagement with what you suggest.

I remember the reaction of a dietitian who looked shocked when I asked why she advised a talkative, extroverted Christian woman to manage her distress through solitary mindfulness and yoga instead of encouraging her to share her emotions and experiences during their clinical encounter or with a trusted friend. She became defensive and said, "Everything I suggested was evidence-based," but evidence-based for whom?

Spirituality is a force meant to grow and mature. Often, a person can revive meaningful religious practices that they dropped earlier in life, which can now support their sense of meaning and growth. Humans often do best when they re-examine earlier practices they were not ready for but are now, or when they integrate new strategies with the old, such as using meditation to engage prayerfully with their faith. They also tend to do better when they connect with like-minded individuals who are pursuing spiritual growth in a similar way. The goal of the practitioner is not to amaze themselves with the latest spiritual practices that worked for someone else.

Consider having a "coffee table" book filled with nature scenes, pets, or travel destinations for someone to browse while waiting. If meeting virtually, share relaxing images along with calming music to start the session with a moment of deep breathing or meditation. If you notice someone becoming emotionally escalated, try to quiet and soften your voice to help them center themselves. Encourage them to take a deep breath, express what's on their mind, or guide them to visualize a calming memory, if you think that could help. You may also ask questions to let them share their thoughts. Spiritual care can be a centering and grounding experience for many, but our follow-up must be tailored to each individual's needs.

The next few pages will include some spiritually enriching practices that dietitians could use in the midst of nutrition counseling if they see the patient needing something more.

## Other complementary spiritual practices to suggest between sessions:[310]

- Play: Use of one's imagination and natural creativity to prevent or resolve emotional/spiritual distress to promote healing and growth.

- Mindfulness: Focus of attention and concentration, a meditation not in emptiness but grounded in God or HP/transformation energy.

- Walking a labyrinth or a sacred path: Heightens spiritual awareness and coping resources for healing.

- Journaling: Writing of events, feelings, experiences or just spontaneous writing for a time. Lowers heart rate and heightens immune function.

- Humor: Laughter releases endorphins, increases the body's ability to heal and heightens the immune system.

- Guided imagery: Directed imagination, creation of visuals, images and events which increase relaxation and well-being.

- Gratitude: Cultivating gratitude, expressing it in writing and or personally, focusing on the positive. Improves sleep, cardiovascular functioning and positive feelings.

- Forgiveness: Forgiving others unblocks spiritual process, lessens tension and anger, helps decrease anxiety and depression.

- Contemplation/centering prayer: Method of prayerful openness. Promotes relaxation, spiritual development and physical healing.

- Breathwork, slow breathing: Increases closeness to God and has positive health benefits.

- Aromatherapy: Using essential oils or other aromas to bring a sense of calm and well-being.

- Poetry: Anything beautiful and awe-inspiring can assist a person to get in touch with deeper needs, desires and sense of transcendent/God. See Food Poetry poems.

- Fasting: Abstaining from all food and drink or restricted menu in order to facilitate faithful responsiveness to God. This is a multi-faith practice.[311]

- String of Beads: Using beads to guide, remind and draw someone to prayer.

# FOOD POETRY

*Strawberrying*

*by May Swensen (1913-1989)*

My hands are murder-red. Many a plump head

drops on the heap in the basket. Or, ripe to bursting

they might be hearts, matching

the blackbirds wing-fleck. Gripped to

need he shrieks his ko-ka-nee in the next field

He's left his peck in some juicy cheeks, when

at first blush and mostly white, they

showed streaks of sweetness to the marauder.

We've picking near the shore this morning, sunny,

a slight wind moving rough-veined leaves

Our hands rumple among. Fingers find by feel

the ready fruit in clusters. Here and there, their squishy wounds . . .
flesh was perfect yesterday . . . June was for gorging

Sweet hearts young & firm before decay

Take only the biggest and not too ripe

A mother calls to he girl and boy, barefoot

In the furrows. Don't step on any in the furrow! Don't!

Change rows. Don't eat too many. Mesmerized

Take only the largesse, the children squat and pull

and pick handfuls of rich scarlets, half for the bucket, half for avid
mouths. Soon whole faces are stained. A Crop this thick begs for
plunder. Ripeness!

From Stacey Harwood, May 1, 2013, saveur.com

*A Miracle for Breakfast*

*by Elizabeth Bishop*

At six o'clock we were waiting for coffee,

waiting for coffee and the charitable crumb

that was going to be served from a certain balcony

– like kings of old, or like a miracle.

It was still dark. One foot of the sun

steadied itself on a long ripple in the river.

The first ferry of the day had just crossed the river.

It was so cold we hoped that the coffee

would be very hot, seeing that the sun

was not going to warm us; and that the crumb

would be a loaf each, buttered, by a miracle.

At seven a man stepped out on the balcony.

He stood for a minute alone on the balcony

looking over our heads toward the river.

A servant handed him the makings of a miracle,

consisting of one lone cup of coffee

and one roll, which he proceeded to crumb,

his head, so to speak, in the clouds–along with the sun.

Was the man crazy? What under the sun

was he trying to do, up there on his balcony!

Each man received one rather hard crumb

which some flicked scornfully into the river,

and, in a cup, one drop of the coffee.

Some of us stood around, waiting for the miracle.

I can tell you what I saw next; it was not a miracle.

A beautiful villa stood in the sun

and from its doors came the smell of hot coffee.

*In front, a baroque white plaster balcony*

*added by birds, who nest along the river,*

*– I saw it with one eye close to the crumb –*

*and galleries and marble chambers. My crumb*

*and mansion, made for me by a miracle,*

*through ages, by insects, birds, and the river*

*working the stone. Every day, in the sun,*

*at breakfast time I sit on my balcony*

*with my feet up, and I drink gallons of coffee.*

*We licked up the crumb and swallowed the coffee.*

*A window across the river caught the sun*

*as if the miracle were working, on the wrong balcony.*

*(A poem about poverty & food in the Great Depression)*

## A String & A Prayer

The practice of making and using a string of beads is over 40,000 years old. It is a practice that creates a tactile connection between our bodies, our senses and our spirits. It can help center us to focus on the divine/transcendent and get out of our own heads of worry. Fossilized shell and bone bead strings (necklaces) were found in Czech Republic showing that the earliest humans used them to adorn themselves, as instruments of prayer, as counting mechanisms, and reminders of important values and needs.

Consider having supplies to share with patients of bead strings of 10 beads on short leather string. Beads could be in colors of foods you want them to remember to consume, like 4 green beads for vegetables, 2 purple for polyphenols, 3 white for calcium-rich foods and yellow for healthy fats.

More than a counting mechanism, they can be tied in a circle, carried in the pocket and used to be a tangible reminder to meditate and pray. In Sanskrit the term *japa-mala* meant *muttering chaplet* which means the beads' function was for recording the number of prayers muttered. Each bead is counted as an individual prayer or mantra. Beads can symbolize a commitment to a spiritual life and self-care practices.

To make a spirit string, take about 10 inches of narrow leather string and 10 beads. (They can be wood, polished stones with holes in the center, seeds etc.) String them and tie them and put them in your pocket.

Practitioners! When you use the following survey with a client to assess their spiritual assets and needs, you can have them fill this out when you start working with them and again when they finish working with you or after a period of care. This is often very helpful for them to see progress.

## SISRI-24 The Spiritual Intelligence Self-Report Inventory

© 2008 D. King Sex (circle one) M F,

The following statements are designed to measure various behaviours, thought processes, and mental characteristics. Read each statement carefully and choose which one of the five possible responses best reflects you by circling the corresponding number. If you are not sure, or if a statement does not seem to apply to you, choose the answer that seems the best. Please answer honestly and make responses based on how you actually are rather than how you would like to be. The five possible responses are:

**0 – Not at all true of me**

**1 – Not very true of me**

**2 – Somewhat true of me**

**3 – Very true of me**

**4 – Completely true of me For each item, circle the one response that most accurately describes you.**

1. I have often questioned or pondered the nature of reality. 0 1 2 3 4

2. I recognize aspects of myself that are deeper than my physical body. 0 1 2 3 4

3. I have spent time contemplating the purpose or reason for my existence. 0 1 2 3 4

4. I am able to enter higher states of consciousness or awareness. 0 1 2 3 4

5. I am able to deeply contemplate what happens after death. 0 1 2 3 4

6. It is difficult for me to sense anything other than the physical and material. 0 1

7. My ability to find meaning and purpose in life helps me adapt to stressful situations. 0 1 2 3 4

8. I can control when I enter higher states of consciousness or awareness. 0 1 2 3 4

9. I have developed my own theories about such things as life, death, reality, and existence. 0 1 2 3 4

10. I am aware of a deeper connection between myself and other people. 0 1 2 3 4

11. I am able to define a purpose or reason for my life. 0 1 2 3 4

12. I am able to move freely between levels of consciousness or awareness. 0 1 2 3 4

13. I frequently contemplate the meaning of events in my life. 0 1 2 3 4

14. I define myself by my deeper, non-physical self. 0 1 2 3 4

15. When I experience a failure, I am still able to find meaning in it. 0 1 2 3 4

16. I often see issues and choices more clearly while in higher states of consciousness/awareness. 0 1 2 3 4

17. I have often contemplated the relationship between human beings and the rest of the universe. 0 1 2 3 4

18. I am highly aware of the nonmaterial aspects of life. 0 1 2 3 4

19. I am able to make decisions according to my purpose in life. 0 1 2 3 4

20. I recognize qualities in people which are more meaningful than their body, personality, or emotions. 0 1 2 3 4

21. I have deeply contemplated whether or not there is some greater power or force (e.g., god, goddess, divine being, higher energy, etc.). 0 1 2 3 4

22. Recognizing the nonmaterial aspects of life helps me feel centered. 0 1 2 3 4

23. I am able to find meaning and purpose in my everyday experiences. 0 1 2 3 4

24. I have developed my own techniques for entering higher states of consciousness or awareness. 0 1 2 3 4

## The Spiritual Intelligence Self-Report Inventory (SISRI-24) Scoring Procedures

Total Spiritual Intelligence Score: Sum all item responses or subscale scores (after accounting for *reverse-coded item).

24 items in total; Range: 0 – 96 4 Factors/Subscales:

I Critical Existential Thinking (CET): Sum items 1, 3, 5, 9, 13, 17, and 21.

7 items in total; range: 0 - 28 II.

II Personal Meaning Production (PMP): Sum items 7, 11, 15, 19, and 23. 5 items in total; range: 0 – 20

III Transcendental Awareness (TA): Sum items 2, 6*, 10, 14, 18, 20, and 22.

7 items in total; range: 0 – 28

Conscious State Expansion (CSE): Sum items 4, 8, 12, 16, and 24. 5 items in total; range: 0 - 20

*Reverse Coding: Item # 6 (response must be reversed prior to summing scores).

Higher scores represent higher levels of spiritual intelligence and/or each capacity.

Permissions for Use of the SISRI is unrestricted so long as it is for academic, educational, or research purposes.

Unlimited duplication of this scale is allowed with full author acknowledgement only. Alterations and/or modifications of any kind are strictly prohibited without author permission.

The author would appreciate a summary of findings from any research which utilizes the SISRI.

Contact details are below. For additional information, please visit http://www.dbking.net/spiritualintelligence/ or e-mail David King at davidking2311@gmail.com

## Spiritual Self-Assessment: Word Pairs

Below you will find seven contrasting pairs of words. Circle the number on the line between the words that best describes how you feel today.

| | | | | | | | | | | | |
|---|---|---|---|---|---|---|---|---|---|---|---|
| fearful | 1 | 2 | 3 | 4 | 5 | 6 | 7 | 8 | 9 | 10 | courageous |
| helpless | 1 | 2 | 3 | 4 | 5 | 6 | 7 | 8 | 9 | 10 | empowered |
| anxious | 1 | 2 | 3 | 4 | 5 | 6 | 7 | 8 | 9 | 10 | At peace |
| alone | 1 | 2 | 3 | 4 | 5 | 6 | 7 | 8 | 9 | 10 | connected |
| despairing | 1 | 2 | 3 | 4 | 5 | 6 | 7 | 8 | 9 | 10 | Hopeful |
| wandering | 1 | 2 | 3 | 4 | 5 | 6 | 7 | 8 | 9 | 10 | Purposeful |
| guilty | 1 | 2 | 3 | 4 | 5 | 6 | 7 | 8 | 9 | 10 | forgiven |
| At Peace With Higher Power/God | 1 | 2 | 3 | 4 | 5 | 6 | 7 | 8 | 9 | 10 | |
| At Peace with yourself | 1 | 2 | 3 | 4 | 5 | 6 | 7 | 8 | 9 | 10 | |
| At peace with family/friends | 1 | 2 | 3 | 4 | 5 | 6 | 7 | 8 | 9 | 10 | |
| At Peace with medical care | 1 | 2 | 3 | 4 | 5 | 6 | 7 | 8 | 9 | 10 | |

Table adapted from resource from National Association of Catholic Chaplains,

https://www.nacc.org/resources/

# A Blank Verbatim Report

**Providers first name:**

I    INFORMATION about the Client: A summary of important information that impacts your supportive care of the patient. Use initials and only information that helps participants understand patient's needs in order to maintain confidentiality.

II    OBSERVATIONS *What you observe in the patient's demeanor and needs on the day of the encounter.*

What are your feelings going into the encounter? *Be as honest with yourself as possible. Notice strong, persistent, over-all feelings or the lack of these.*

**What do you observe about the setting, the person?**

III    VERBATIM P = Provider CL = Client

Example: Try to remember as clear as you can the actual dialogue between you and the client. Also note your own feelings, reactions and your own inner dialogue while you worked with the client. Be as honest as you can so you can learn about yourself as you provide care. Use P for Provider, CL for the client: Number the responses.

P1:

CL1:

P2:

CL2:

## V. EVALUATION & SUPERVISION

Why did you choose this nutrition counseling encounter?

What are you learning as you record this encounter?

What do you learn about human nature, spirituality, and the Sacred in this encounter?

What social or cultural forces are at work?

Where do you want supervision or input from peers?

Verbatim adapted from verbatim form from https://www.apchaplains.org/

# Verbatim Reflection

**1**

### Why did I pick this interaction for the verbatim?

What did I like about this interaction? Where did I struggle, feel uncomfortable, not be as helpful as I would hope? What did I say, do or feel? Where do I hope to learn from?

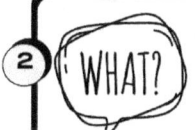

**2**

### What is my style of interaction?

Do I interact empathetically or do I tend to be intellectual? Did I do anything to keep the interaction superficial? Was what I said and did congruent? What would I do differently next time?

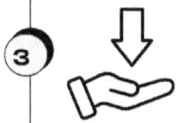

**3**

### What did the person seem to need from me?

What did the person need emotionally and spiritually from me? Are they spiritually distressed or grieving? How do they recharge themselves or do they?

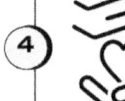

**4**

### How would I describe the spiritual issue/need or concern?

Review the spirituality checklist from Chapter 3. How would I describe their need? Did I address this or utilize it for promoting their health? Who should address this need?

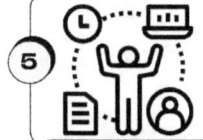

**5**

### What spiritual resources would be helpful for this person?

Did a spiritual image, theme or text come to my mind? Did I share that and what was the outcome? Did I gauge my use of a spiritual tool on what I heard from the patient?

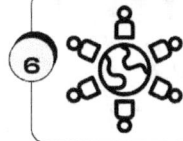

**6**

### What cultural needs does this person present?

Are there any cultural implications that will impact my supportive lifestyle care of this patient? Do I need to review the information about other religious traditions next time?

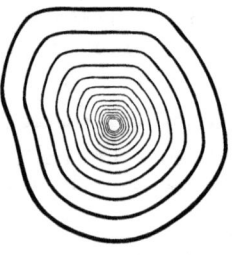

*References*

# Endnotes

1    Salmasy D, *The Rebirth of the Clinic: An Introduction to Spirituality in Healthcare* (Georgetown University Press, 2006) p. 40.

2    Teixeira Pinto C, Guedes L, Pinto S, Nunes R, "Spiritual intelligence: a scoping review on the gateway to mental health," *Global Health Action*, 17, 2362310 (2023).

3    Ibid.

4    Sahebalzamani M, Farahani H, Abasi R, Talebi M, "The relationship between spiritual intelligence with psychological well-being and purpose in life of nurses," *Iranian J of Nursing and Midwifery Research*, Jan-Feb 2012, 18, 1 (2013): 38–41.

5    Russo-Netzer Pninit, "Building Bridges, Forging new Frontiers: Meaning-Making in Action," *Social Sciences* 12, 574 (2023).

6    Ibid.

7    Errasti-Ibarrondo B, Jordán JA, Díez-Del-Corral MP, Arantzamendi M. "van Manen's phenomenology of practice: How can it contribute to nursing?" *Nurs Inq.* 26(1) (2019):e12259

8    Cohen B, Hyman S, Rosenberg L, Larson E, "Frequency of patient contact with health care personnel and visitors: implications for infection prevention," *Jt Comm J Qual Patient Saf.* 38(12) (2012): 560–5.

9    https://www.hhs.gov/guidance/sites/default/files/hhs-guidance-documents/R11272CP.pdf

10    Noland D, Sudha R, "Academy of Nutrition and Dietetics: Revised 2019 Standards of Practice and Standards of Professional Performance for Registered Dietitian Nutritionists (Competent, Proficient, and expert) in Nutrition in Integrative and Functional Medicine," *Journal of the Academy of Nutrition Dietetics*, June 119, 6, 1019–1036.

11    Kris Etherton P, Akabas S, Bales C, Bistrian B, Braun L, Edwards M, et al. "The need to advance nutrition education in the training of healthcare professionals and recommended research to evaluate, implement and effectiveness," April 9, 99, 5 (2014): 1153S-1166S

12    Pinto Teixeira, "Spiritual intelligence," 2024.

13  Collins, J, "The Utilization of Spirituality in Occupational Therapy: Beliefs, Practices & Barriers," Occup Ther Health Care. 2002;14(3-4):73-92. doi: 10.1080/J003v14n03_05.

14  Hwalla N, Koleilat M, "Dietetic practice: the past, present and future, La Revue de Sante de la Mediterranee orientale," 10, 6, (2004).

15  Skiadas PK Lascaratos JG, "Dietetics in ancient Greek philosophy: Plato's concepts of healthy diet," European Journal of Clinical Nutrition, 55, 7 (2001): 532–7.

16  Nagy A, McMahon A, Tapesll L, Deane, F, "The Therapeutic relationship between a client and dietitian: A Systematic integrative review of empirical literature," Nutrition & Dietetics, 79: (2022): 303–348.

17  Gesser-Edelsberg A, Birman Y, "Does the transformation of dietitians from counseling to therapy also apply to the physical and therapeutic environment? A case study of Israeli Practice," J Acad Nutri Diet, 118 (2018):1047–1056.

18  Swan W, Vivanti A, Hakel-Smith N, Hotson B, Orrevall Y, Trostler N, Howarter K, Papoutsakis C, "Nutrition Care Process and Model Update: Toward Realizing People-Centered Care and Outcomes management," Journal of the Academy of Nutrition and Dietetics, Dec, 117, 12 (2017): 2003–2014.

19  Hackert AN, Kniskern MA, Beasley TM, "Academy of Nutrition and Dietetics: Revised 2020 Standards of Practice and Standards of Professional Performance for Registered Dietitian Nutritionist in Eating Disorders," J Acad Nutr Diet Nov, 120, 11 (2020): 1902–1919.

20  Ibid.

21  Yang w, Fu Y, "Level of empathy among dietitians: a pilot study," Nutrition Diet. 75 (2018): 411–417.

22  McSherry W, Ross L, "Dilemmas of spiritual assessment: considerations for nursing practice," Journal of Advanced Nursing 38, 5 (2002): 479.

23  Jarden A, Roache A, "What is Wellbeing?" Inter J Environ Res Public Health, 20 (2023): 5006.

24   Lomas T, VanderWeele T, "The Garden and the Orchestra: Generative Metaphors for Conceptualizing the complexities of Well-Being," Int J Environ Res Public Health 19 (2022): 14544.

25   Health Equity & Policy Lab at the University of Pennsylvania, https://www.healthequityandpolicylab.com/human-flourishing

26   Lomas & VanderWeele, "The Garden and the Orchestra" 2022.

27   Kopacz M, Morley SW, Wozniak B, Simons KV, Bishop TM, Garland Vance C, "Religious Well-Being and Suicide Ideation in Veterans-An Exploratory Study," Pastoral Psychology, 65(4) (2016): 481–491.

28   Idler EL, George LK, Cohesiveness and coherence: Religion and the health of the elderly (New York: Garland Publishing, 1998).

29   Kopacz M et al., "Religious Well-Being and Suicide Ideation in Veterans," 2016.

30   Hancock REE, Bonner G, Hollingdale S, Madden AM, "If you listen to me properly, I feel good': a qualitative examination of patient experiences of dietetic consultations," Journal Human Nutrition & Dietetics, 25 (2012): 275–284.

31   Noland D, Raj S, "Academy of Nutrition and Dietetics: Revised 2019 Standards of Practice and Standards of Professional Performance for Registered Dietitian Nutritionists," 2019.

32   Pen-Keller S (1983-1984) "The World Health Assembly Debates the Spiritual Dimension", from The Spirit of Global Health: The World Health Organization and the Spiritual Dimension of Health, 1946-2021, Peng-Keller Oxford University Press.

33   World Health Organization, 1983.

34   Pen-Keller S (1983-1984) "The World Health Assembly Debates the Spiritual Dimension", from The Spirit of Global Health: The World Health Organization and the Spiritual Dimension of Health, 1946-2021, Peng-Keller Oxford University Press.

35   Joint Commission, July 19, 2022, Spiritual Beliefs & Preferences, Critical Access Hospital Manual, Chapter Provisions of Care, Treatment & Services.

36    National Consensus Project for Quality Palliative Care, 2018, Clinical Practice Guidelines for Quality Palliative Care, 4th edition. Richmond, VA: National Coalition for Hospice and Palliative Care; 2018.

37    Hatala A, "Towards a BioPsychosocial-Spiritual Approach in Health Psychology: Exploring Theoretical Orientations and Future Directions," Journal of Spirituality in Mental Health, 2013, 14:4, 256–276.

38    Sulmasy DP. "A biopsychosocial-spiritual model for the care of patients at the end of life," Gerontologist. 42 Spec No 3 (2002):24–33.

39    Mittelmark, M, Bauer, G, "Salutogenesis as a theory, as an orientation and as the sense of coherence, the Handbook for Salutogenesis," 2nd Edition, Cham Springer, NCBI Bookshelf (2022).

40    Collins, J, "The Utilization of Spirituality in Occupational Therapy: Beliefs, Practices & Barriers," 2000.

41    Augustine, of Hippo, 354-430, Saint, Confessions, Mount Vernon: Peter Pauper Press.

42    Eichstaedt J, Zhao Y, Valillant G, Newberg A, "The overview effect: Awe and self-transcendent experience in space flight," Psychology of Consciousness: Theory, Research, and Practice, 3(2) (2016): 145.

43    Penman J, "Cognitive and Behavioral Changes Arising from Spirituality," Journal of Religion and Health 60 (2021): 4082-4096.

44    Oishi S, Westgate EC, "A Psychologically Rich Life: Beyond Happiness and Meaning," Psychol Rev, 129 (2022): 790-811.

45    Frankl VE, 1963.

46    Russo-Netzer P, "Building Bridges, Forging new Frontiers," 2023.

47    Ibid.

48    Warpeha A, Harris J, "Combining Traditional and nontraditional approaches to nutrition counseling, Perspectives in Practice," Journal of the American Dietetic Association, 93,7 (1993): 797-800.

49    Dittmann k, Freedman M, Beddow A, Waldrop J, "Body awareness, eating attitudes and spiritual beliefs of women who practice yoga: a case for

recovery," Journal of Dietetic Association, Sept, Suppl 3 108, 9 (2008).

50  Chester D, Himburg S, Weatherspoon L, "Spirituality of African-American women: correlations to health promoting behaviors," Journal of National Black Nursing Association, July, 17, 1 (2006): 1-8.

51  Brown E, Bearden R, Roberts R, O'Donohue, "7 Stepping Stones-Using spirituality to enhance nutrition and wellness programs for Jesse Brown Veterans Administration medical Center," Journal of the Acad of Nutrition and Dietetics, Supple 3 112, 9 (2012).

52  Morris A, Biggerstaff, Lycett D, "Capturing whole person care," Journal of Renal Care, 42, 2, (2016): 71–72.

53  Gesser-Edelsburg A, Birman Y, "Does the Transformation of dietitians from counseling to therapy also apply to physical and therapeutic environment? A case study of Israeli Practice," Journal of Acad of Nutrition Dietetics, 118, 6, (2018): 1047–1056.

54  Lycett D, Garvey S, Patel R, "A survey regarding the role of UK dietitians in spiritual care," J Human Nutr Diet, 37 (2024): 749-761.

55  Engquist DE, Short-DeGraff, Gliner J, Oltjenbruns K, "Occupational therapist' beliefs and practices with regard to spirituality and therapy," The American Journal of Occupational Therapy, 51, 3, (1997): 173-180.

56  Heyen A, Levine A Muse-Burke J, Krokus M, Bodzio J, "RDN's Intrinsic Religiosity and Continuing Education Predict their Orientation Towards Religious/Spiritually Integrated Practice," Journal of the Academy of Nutrition & Dietetics, Sept, Suppl 1 Abstracts 121, 9 (2021).

57  Engquist DE, Short-DeGraff, Gliner J, Oltjenbruns K, "Occupational therapist' beliefs and practices with regard to spirituality and therapy," The American Journal of Occupational Therapy, 51, 3 (1997): 173-180.

58  Heyen, "RDN's Intrinsic Religiosity and Continuing Education Predict their Orientation Towards Religious/Spiritually Integrated Practice," 2021.

59  King U, The search for spirituality. Our global quest for meaning and fulfillment (Canterbury Press, 2009).

60    Nita M, "Spirituality in Health Studies: Competing Spiritualities & Elevated Status of Mindfulness," Journal of Relig Health, 50, 5 (2019): 1605-1618.

61    Ibid.

62    Hilsman, G, 2024, personal conversation with author.

63    Frankl, V. Man's Search for Meaning (Beacon Press, 1959).

64    Enquist, "Occupational therapist' beliefs and practices with regard to spirituality and therapy," 173-180.

65    Gavaza P, Bhaktidevi R, Johnston Taylor E, 2022, "Perspectives about spiritual care in pharmacy practice: a community-based survey," Innov Pharm, 13,4, 10.24926/iip.v13i4.5098.

66    UKCC, 1984, Code of Professional Conduct for Nurses, Midwives and health Visitors, UKCC, London.

67    Egan M, DeLatt MD, 1997, "The Implicit Spirituality of occupational therapy practice," Canadian Journal of Occupational Therapy, 64,1, 95-101.

68    Gavaza P, Rawal B, Johnston Taylor E, 2022, "Perspectives about Spiritual Care in Pharmacy Practice: A Community-based Survey," Innov Pharm, 13, 4.

69    Harrad R, Cosentino C, Keasley R, Sulla F, 2019, "Spiritual care in nursing: an overview of the measures used to assess spiritual care provision and related factors amongst nurses," Acta Bilmed for Health Professions, Vol 90, S. 4:44-55.

70    Ibid.

71    Meyer CL, 2003, "How effectively are Nurse Educators preparing Students to Provide Spiritual Care?" Nurse Educ, July 1, 28, 4, 185-90.

72    Kytoko JJ, Knight SJ, "Body, mind, Spirit: Towards the integration of religiosity and spirituality in cancer quality of life research," Psychooncology 8, 439-450 1999.

73    Emblen, 1992, Religion and spirituality defined according to current use in nursing literature, Journal Professional Nursing 8, 41-47

74    Hilsman GJ, Spiritual Care in common Terms (Jessica Kingsley Publishing, 2017) p.47.

75    Emblen, 1992, "Religion and spirituality defined according to current use in nursing literature," Journal Professional Nursing 8, 41-47.

76    Ebotabe Arrey A, Bilsen J, Patrick L, Deschepper R, 2016, "Spirituality/ religiosity: A cultural and psychological resource among sub-Saharan African migrant women with HIV/AIDS in Belgium," published online doi. org/10.137/journal.pone0159488

77    Ishaq, B, Ostby L, Johannessen, A, 2021, "Muslim religiosity and health outcomes: A cross-sectional study among Muslims in Norway," SSM Popul Health, Sept, 15, 100843.

78    Salmasy D, The Rebirth of the Clinic: An Introduction to Spirituality in Healthcare (Georgetown University Press, 2006) p. 22.

79    Baldacchino, D, (2015) "Spiritual Care Education of Health Care Professionals," Conference Report, Journal of Religions, 6, 594-613.

80    Burnard p, 1988, "The spiritual needs of atheists and agnostics," The Professional Nurse, Dec, 130-132.

81    Narayanasmy, A (1999) "Asset: A Model of actioning spirituality and spiritual care education and training in nursing," Nurse Education Today, May; 19(4) 274-28534.

82    Colliton M, The Spiritual Dimension of Nursing, Clinical Nursing (Macmillan, 1981).

83    Mische P 1982 "Toward a global spirituality," In Mische P, ed Whole Earth Papers, East Grange NJ Global Education Association No 16.

84    Legere T, 1984 "A spirituality for today," Studies in Formative Spirituality 5 3: 375-385.

85    Bradshaw A, Lighting the lamp: the spiritual dimension of nursing care (Scutari, 1994).

86    Granstrom SI 1985 "Spiritual nursing care for oncology patients," Topics in Clinical Nursing 7, 1, 39-45.

87    Soeken KL, Carson VJ, 1987, "Responding to the spiritual needs of the chronically ill," Nursing Clinics of North America 22 (3) 603-611.

88  Narayanasmy A, "Asset: A Model of actioning spirituality and spiritual care education and training in nursing," 1999.

89  Kurtz E, 1990, "The spirituality of William James: A Lesson from Alcoholics anonymous," Presented at the American Psychological Association 98th Annual Conference, Boston, MA, USA.

90  Kurtz E, The Spirituality of Imperfection (Bantam, 1992).

91  DiReda J, Gonsalvez J, (2016) "The Role of Spirituality in Treating Substance Use Disorders," Journal of Clinical Psychiatry, 6, 4.

92  Salmasy D, The Rebirth of the Clinic: An Introduction to Spirituality in Healthcare (Georgetown University Press, 2006) p. 22.

93  Fowler, J. W., & Dell, M. L. (2006). "Stages of Faith From Infancy Through Adolescence: Reflections on Three Decades of Faith Development Theory." In E. C. Roehlkepartain, P. E. King, L. Wagener, & P. L. Benson (Eds.), The handbook of spiritual development in childhood and adolescence (pp. 34–45).

94  Baltes, 1998 as cited in Mallery, 2022.

95  Kohlberg, L. (1985). Kohlberg's Stages of Moral Development. In Crain, W.C., Ed., Theories of Development, Prentice-Hall, London, 118-136.

96  Margela and Steger, 2016 as cited in Mallery et al., 2022.

97  McCullough, M. E., & Willoughby, B. L. B. (2009). "Religion, self-regulation, and self-control: Associations, explanations, and implications," Psychological Bulletin, 135(1), 69–93. https://doi.org/10.1037/a0014213

98  Tsai, Miao & Seppala, 2007 as cited in McCullough & Willoughby, 2009.

99  Azari, NP, Missimer J & Seitz RJ, 2005, "Religious Experience and Emotion: Evidence for distinctive cognitive neural patterns," International Journal for the Psychology of Religion, 15, 263-281.

100  McCullough and Willoughby, 2009.

101  Cohen AB, 2003, "Religion, likelihood of action and the morality of mentality," International Journal for the Psychology of Religion, 13, 273-285

102  Bushra, 2021.

103 Lycett, D & Patel, R, Spiritual Care within Dietetic Practice: A Systematic Literature Review, 2023. Journal of Religion and Health, 62, 2, 1223–1250.

104 Gibbs, K.E. & Bamitt, R. (1999). "Occupational therapy and the self-care needs of Hindu elders," British Journal of Occupational Therapy, 62, 100-106.

105 Bushra I, Lars O, Asbjorn J, 2021, "Muslim religiosity and health outcomes: A Cross-sectional study among Muslims in Norway," SSM Popul Health, Sept 15, Published online.

106 Tey, SD, Park MS, Golden KJ, 2018, "Religiosity and healthy lifestyle behaviors in Malaysian Muslims: The mediating role of subjective well-being and self-regulation," Journal of Religion and Health, 57, 6, 2050.

107 Kang Y, Strecher V, Kim E, Falk E, 2019, "Purpose in Life-Conflict Related Neural responses during health decision making," Health Psychol, June 38, 6, 545-552.

108 Boylan JM, Biggano C, Shaffer J, Wilson C, Vagnini K, Masters K, 2023 "Do Purpose in Life and Social Support Mediate the Association between Religiousness/Spirituality and Mortality? Evidence from the MIDUS National Sample," Int J Environ Res Public Health 20, 6112.

109 Berkowitz L, Mateo C, Salazar C, et al., 2023 "Healthy Eating a Potential Mediator of Inverse Association Between Purpose in Life and Waist Circumference: Emerging Evidence from US and Chilean Cohorts," Int J Environ Res Public Health, 20, 7099.

110 Steptoe A, Fancourt D 2019, "Leading a meaningful life at older ages and its relationship with social engagement, prosperity, health, biology and time use," Pro Natl Acad Sci USA, 116, 1207-1212.

111 Berkowitz, 2023.

112 Morozink JA, Friedman EM, Co CI, Ryff CD, 2010, "Socioeconomic and psychosocial predictors of interleukin-6 in the MIDUS national sample," Health Psychol 29, 626-635.

113 Cole SW, Levine ME, Arevalo JMG, Ma, J, Weir DR, Crimmins EM, 2015, "Loneliness, eudaimonia and the human conserved transcriptional response to adversity," Psychoneuroendocrinology 62, 11-17.

114    Guimon AJ, Shiba K, Kim ES, Kubzansky LD 2022, Sense of purpose in life and inflammation in healthy older adults: A longitudinal study, Psychoneuroendocrinology 141,105746.

115    Guimond AJ, Shiba K, Kim ES, Kubzansky LD,2022, Sense of purpose in life and inflammation in healthy older adults: A longitudinal study. Psychoneuroendocrinology. Jul; 141:105746.

116    Dalmida SG, Holstad MN, DiIorio C Laderman G, 2011, Spiritual well-being and health related quality of life among African American women with HIV/AIDS, Appl Res Qual Life, Jun; 6, 2, 139-157.

117    Chaix R, Fagny M, Cosin-Tomas M, Alvarez-Lopez M, Lemee L, Regnault B, Davidson RJ, LutzA, Kailman P, 2020, Differential DNA methylation in experienced meditators after an intensive day of mindfulness-based practice: Implications for immune-related pathways, Feb 84:36-44.

118    Kaliman P, Alvarez-Lopez M, Cosin-Tomas, Rosenkranz M, Lutz A, Davidson R, 2014, Rapid changes in histone deacetylases and inflammatory gene expression in expert meditators, Feb 40, 96-107.

119    Tsenkova VK, Love GD, Singer BH, Ryff CD, 2007, Socioeconomic status and psychological well-being predict cross-time change in glycosylated hemoglobin in older women without diabetes, Psychosom Med, 69,777-784.

120    Rasmussen NH, Smith SA, Maxson JA, Bernard ME, Cha SS, Agerter DC, Shah ND, 2013 Association of HbA1c with emotion regulation, intolerance of uncertainty and purpose in life in type 2 diabetes mellitus, Prim Care Diabetes, 7,213-221.

121    Hafez D, Heisler M, Choe H Ankuda CK, Winkelman T, Kullgren JI, 2018, Association between purpose in life and glucose control among older adults, Ann Behav Med, 52, 309-318.

122    Cohen R Bavishi C, Rozanski A, 2016, Purpose in life and its relationship to all-cause mortality and cardiovascular events: A meta-analysis. Psychosom Med, 78,122-133.

123    Sutin DAR, Luchetti M, Aschwanden D, Stephan Y, Sesker AA, Teracciano A, 2023, A sense of meaning and purpose in life and risk of incident dementia:

new data and meta-analysis, Arch gerontol geriatr, 105, 104847.

124    Bamonti P, Lombardi S, Buberstein, King D, VanOrden K, 2016, Spirituality Attenuates the Association Between Depression Symptom Severity and Meaning in Life, Aging Ment Health, May;20, 5, 494-499

125    Fox M, 1994, The Reinvention of work: A New vision of Livelihood for our Time, Harper San Francisco, San Francisco, CA

126    Bożek A, Nowak PF, Blukacz M., 2020, The Relationship Between Spirituality, Health-Related Behavior, and Psychological Well-Being. Front Psychol, Aug 14;11:1997

127    Duke N, 2021, Type 2 diabetes self-management: spirituality, coping and responsibility, Journal of Research in Nursing, 26,8, 743-760

128    Kaleyci V, Levine A, Krokus M, Bodzio J, 2021, Spirituality Predicts body appreciation, which is related to higher quality of life, Journal of the Academy Nutrition Dietetics, suppl 1 121, 9, A61

129    Homan K, Boyatzis C, 2009, Body Image in Older Adults: Links with Religion and Gender, J Adult Dev. 16: 230-238

130    Penman F, 2021, Cognitive and behavioral changes arising from spirituality, Journal of Religion and Health, 60,4082-4096

131    Macquarrie J, 1972, Existentialism Penguin, Harmondsworth

132    Kass, J. D., Friedman, R., Lesserman, J., Zutter meister, P., & Benson, H. "Health outcomes and a new index of spiritual experience," Journal for the Scientific Study of Religion, 30(2) (1991): 203-211.

133    Hamilton & Kroska, 2018.

134    Exline j, Homolka S, Harriot V, 2016, Divine struggles: Links with body image concerns, binging and compensatory behaviors around eating, Mental Health, Religion & Culture, 19, 1, 8-22.

135    Esperandio M, Viacava J, Franco R, Pargament K, Exline J, 2022, Brazilian Adaptation and Validation of the Religious and Spiritual Struggles (RSS) Scale-Extended and Short Version, Religions, 13, 282.

136    Hilsman, 2017.

137     M Klimasinski et.al, 2022 Spiritual Distress and spiritual needs of chronically Ill patients in Poland: A Cross-sectional Study, Intern J Environ Res and Public Health, 19, 5512.

139     Pagament KI, Koenig HG, Tarakeshwar N & Hahn J, 2001, Religious struggle as a predictor of mortality among medically ill elderly patients; A two-year longitudinal study, Archives of Internal Medicine, 161,1881-1885.

140     Oluwaseyi O. Isehunwa, E, Warner, T, Spiegelman D, Huang T, Shelley Tworoger, S, , Kent B, Shields A, 2021, Religion, spirituality and diurnal rhythms of salivary cortisol and dehydroepiandrosterone in postmenopausal women, Comprehensive Psychoneuroendocrinology, Volume 7, 100064.

141     Koenig HG, Pargament KI, Nielsen J, 1998, Religious coping and health status in medically ill hospitalized older adults, Journal of Nervous and mental disease, 186, 513-521.

142     Lycett & Patel, 2023.

143     Riazi A, Pickup J, Bradley C, 2004, Daily Stress and Glycemic Control in Type 1 diabetes, individual differences in magnitude, direction and timing of stress-reactivity, Diabetes Research & Clinical Practice, 66,3, 237-244.

144     Ano G, Pargament KI, 2013, Predictors of spiritual struggles: an exploratory study, Mental Health Religion and Culture, 16, 419-434.

145     Wood BT, Worthington E L Jr, Exline JJ, Yali A, Aten AM, McMinn MR,2010, Development, refinement, and psychometric properties of the attitudes toward God scale, Psychology of Religion and Spirituality, 2, 148-167.

146     Grubbs JB, Exline JJ, Wilt JA, Pargament KI, 2016, Personality, Religious and Spiritual Struggles, and Well-Being Psychology of Religion and Spirituality 8, 4.

147     Grubbs JB, Exline JJ, Campbell WK, 2013, I deserve better and God knows it! Psychological entitlement as a robust predictor of anger at God. Psychology of Religion and Spirituality, 5, 192-200.

148     Van Leeuwen R, Tiesinga L, Post D, Jochemsen H, 2006, Spiritual Care: Implications for nurses' professional responsibility, Journal of Clinical Nursing, 15,7, 875-884.

149    Bhatnagar S, Gielen J, Satija A, Singh S, Noble S, Chaturvedi S, 2017, Signs of Spiritual Distress and its Implications for Practice in Indian Palliative Care, Indian J Palliative Care, Jul-Sept, 23, 3, 306-311.

150    Exline J, Homolka S, Harriott V, 2015, Divine struggles: links with body image concerns, binging, and compensatory behaviors around eating, Mental health, religion and culture, 19, 1, 8-22.

151    Abramowitz, J, Huppet J, Cohen A, Tolin D, Cahill S, 2002, Religious Obsessions and compulsions in a non-clinical sample: The Penn Inventory of Scrupulosity (PIOS), Behaviour Research and Therapy, 40, 824-838.

152    Richards PS, Smith MH, Berrett ME, O'Grady KA, Bartz JD, 2009, A theistic spiritual treatment for women with eating disorders, Journal of Clinical Psychology: IN Session, 75, 172-184

153    Exline et al., 2015.

154    Exline et al., 2015.

155    Sharma R, Astrow A, Texeira K, Sulmasy D, 2012, The Spiritual Needs Assessment for Patients (SNAP): Development and Validation of a Comprehensive Instrument to Asses Unmet Spiritual Needs, Journal of Pain and Symptom Management, 44, 1, July.

156    Wolfelt, A. D., Wolfelt, A., & Duvall, K. J. (2009). Healing your grieving body: 100 physical practices for mourners. Companion Press.

157    Mughal S, Azhar Y, Mahon M, Siddiqui W, 2024, Grief Reaction and Prolonged Grief Disorder, No 14, In Stat Pearls, Treasure Island FL, Stat Pearls Publishing.

158    Wolfelt A, 2006, Companioning the Bereaved, Companion Press, Fort Collins, CO.

159    Wolfelt A, 2007, Living in the Shadow of the Ghosts of Grief: Step into the light, Companion Press, Fort Collins, CO.

160    Mughal, 2024.

161    Lundorff M, Bonanno GA, Johannsen M, O'Connor M., 2020, Are there gender differences in prolonged grief trajectories? A registry-sampled cohort

study. J Psychiatr Res. Oct; 129: 168-175.

162    Mughal, 2024.

163    Doka K, 2009, Disenfranchised Grief, Bereavement Care, 18, 3

164    Haupt A, 2023, https://time.com/6275929/weight-gain-body-grief/

165    Wolfelt & Duvall, 2009.

166    Wolfelt, 2007.

167    Ibid.

168    Ibid.

169    Young M, Benjamin B, Wallis C, "The mortality of widowers," Lancet, 1963, 13:454-456.

170    Edmondson D, Newman JD, Whang W, Davidson KW, 2013, Emotional triggers in myocardial infarction: do they matter? Eur Heart J, Jan 34, 4, 300-306.

171    Mughal, 2024.

172    Irwin M, Daniels M, Risch S, Bloom E, Weiner H, 1988, Plasma Cortisol and natural killer cell activity during bereavement, Bilo Psychiatry, 24,173-178.

173    Buckley T, Sunari D, Marshall A, Bartrop R, Mckinley S, Tofler G, 2012, Physiological Correlates of bereavement and the impact of bereavement Interventions, Dialogues in Clinical Neuroscience, 14:2, 129-139.

174    Nicolson NA, 2004, childhood parental loss and cortisol levels in adult men, Psychoneuroendocrinology, 29, 1012-1018.

175    Breier A, 1989, Experimental approaches to human stress research: assessment of neurobiological mechanisms of stress in volunteers and psychiatric patients, Bil Psychiatry, 26, 438-462.

176    Kanfer R, Lord J, Phillips A, 2011, Neutrophil function and cortisol: DHEAS ratio in bereaved older adults, Brain Behav Immun 25, 1182-1186.

177    Schleifer SJ, Keller SE, Camerino M, Thornton JC, Stein M, 1983 suppression of lymphocytes stimulation following bereavement, JAMA, 250, 374-377.

178   Gerra G, Nonti D, Panerai A, 2003, Long-term immune endocrine effects of bereavement: relationships with anxiety levels and mood, Psychiatry Res, 121, 145-158.

179   Gerra G, Nonti D, Panerai A, 2003, Long-term immune endocrine effects of bereavement: relationships with anxiety levels and mood, Psychiatry Res, 121, 145-158.

180   Pore N, Burly M, 2012, When a broken heart is real: Takotsubo cardiomyopathy, Nurse Pract, Oc, 10, 37, 10, 48-52.

181   Goodkin, Feaster DJ, Asthana D, 1998, Bereavement support group intervention is longitudinally associated with salutary effects on the CD4 cell count and number of physician visits, Clin Diagn Lab Immunol, 5:382-391.

182   Johnson C, 2002, Nutritional Considerations for Bereavement and Coping with grief, J Nutr Health Aging May, 6, 3, 171-176.

183   Johnson CS, 2002, Nutritional considerations for bereavement and coping with grief, J Nutr Health aging, May 6, 3, 171-176.

184   Fagundes C, Wu E, 2021, Biological Mechanisms Underlying Widowhood's Health consequences; does diet play a role? Comprehensive Psychoneuroendocrinology, 7, 100058.

185   J.K. Kiecolt-Glaser, C.P. Fagundes, R. Andridge, J. Peng, W.B. Malarkey, D. Habash, M.A. Belury, 2017, Depression, daily stressors and inflammatory responses to high-fat meals: when stress overrides healthier food choices, Mol. Psychiatr. 22 3, 476–482.

186   Fagundes C, Wu E, 2021, Biological Mechanisms Underlying Widowhood's Health consequences; does diet play a role? Comprehensive Psychoneuroendocrinology, 7, 100058

187   Wolfelt, 2009.

188   Wolfelt A, Duvall K, https://www.centerforloss.com/2023/12/healing-grieving-body-physical-practices-mourners/Online article from book, Healing your Grieving Body, Companion Press, Fort Collins, CO

189   Carried Grief Inventory and Loss Inventory from Living in the Shadow of

the Ghosts of Grief, Step into the Light, reconcile old losses and open the door to infinite joy and love, 2007, Alan Wolfelt, PhD, Companion Press, Fort Collins, CO

190   From Wolfelt. 2007.

191   Lycett & Patel, 2023.

192   Hamilton & Kroska, 2018, as cited by Lycett & Patel, 2023.

193   Ibid.

194   Balboni TA, Vanderwerkee LC, Block SD, Paulk ME, Lathan CS, Peteet, JR, Prigerson HG, 2007, Religiousness and spiritual support among advanced cancer patients and associations with end-of-life treatment preferences and quality of life, Journal of clinical Oncology, 25, 5, 55-560.

195   Pearce M, Coan A, Herndon J, Koenig H, Abernethy A, 2012, Unmet Spiritual Care needs impact emotional and spiritual well-being in advanced cancer patients, support Care Cancer, 20: 2269-2276.

196   Astrow AB, Wexler A, Texeira K, He MK, Sulmasy DP 2007 Is failure to meet spiritual needs associated with cancer patients' perceptions of quality of care and their satisfaction with care? Journal of clinical Oncology, 25, 36, 5753-5757.

197   Balboni MJ, Sullivan A, Amobi A, Phelps A, Gorman DP, Zollfrank A, Balboni TA, 2013, Why is spiritual care infrequent at the end of life? Spiritual care perceptions among patients, nurses and physicians and the role of training, Journal of clinical Oncology 31,4, 461-467.

198   Giese-Davis J, Collie K, Rancourt KMS, Neri E, Kramermer, 2011, Decrease in depression symptoms is associated with longer survival in patients with metastatic breast cancer, a secondary analysis, J Clin Oncology, 29 413-420.

199   Puchalski C, 2000, Taking a spiritual history allows clinicians to understand patients more fully, J Palliative Med, 3, 129-137.

200   Anandarajah G, Hight E, 2001, Spirituality and Medical Practice: Using the Hope Questions as a practical tool for spiritual assessment, Am Fam Physician 63,81-8, 89.

201    LaRocca-Pitts, M. (2024). The bidimensional spirit and mattering: A continuum of spiritual care interventions. Spirituality in Clinical Practice. Advance online publication. https://doi.org/10.1037/scp0000377

202    Lycett, "Spiritual Care and Dietetic Practice–A call beyond cultural competency". www.bda.uk.com/resource/spiritual-care-and-dietetic-practice-a-call-beyond-cultural-competency.html

203    McPherson, 2015, The History of the Hippocratic Oath, https://absn.northeastern.edu/blog/the-history-of-the-hippocratic-oath/

204    Academy of Nutrition and Dietetics, 2018, Code of Ethics for the Nutrition and Dietetics Profession, https://www.eatrightpro.org/practice/code-of-ethics/code-of-ethics-for-the-nutrition-and-dietetics-profession

205    Wechkin H, Macauley R, Menzel P, Reagan P, Simmers N, Quill T, 2023, "Clinical Guidelines for Voluntarily Stopping Eating and Drinking," Journal of Pain and Symptom Management, 66, 5, November, e625-e631

206    Ortiz G, 2016, The Ethics of voluntarily stopping eating and drinking, The National Catholic Bioethics Quarterly, Winter, 607-617.

207    Ibid.

208    Meier D, Myers H, Muskin P, 1999, When a Patient Requests Help Committing Suicide, Generations, 23, Spring, 67

209    Chochinov HM, Hassard T, McClement S, Hack T, Krisjanson L, et al, 2008, The Patient Dignity Inventory: A Novel Way of Measuring Dignity-Related Distress in Palliative Care, Journal of Pain and Symptom Management, 36, 6, 559-571

210    McDermott P, 2019, Patient Dignity Question: feasible, dignity-conserving intervention in a rural hospice, Canadian Family Physician, 65, November, 812-819

211    Columbia Narrative medicine, About narrative medicine (New York, NY, 2019).

212    McDermott P, 2019, 812-819.

213    Chocchinov H, 2007, Dignity and the Essence of Medicine: the ABC and D of Dignity Conserving Care, BMJ, 28, 335, 184-187

214    Salmasy D, 2006.

215    Swihart D, Yarrarapu SN, Martin R, 2023, Cultural Religious Competence in Clinical Practice, NCBI Bookshelf, National Library of Medicine, Nation Institutes of Health, Treasure Island, Fl, StatPearls Publishing Jan 2024.

216    Deleyto-Seldas N, Efeyan A. The mTOR-Autophagy Axis and the Control of Metabolism. Front Cell Dev Biol. 2021 Jul 1;9:655731. doi: 10.3389/fcell.2021.655731.

217    Yang, 2022.

218    Facts from El-Zibdeh N, 2009, Understanding Muslim Fasting Practices, 2009, Today's Dietitian, 11,8, 56.

219    Facts summarized from Subramanian K, Mahadevan S, Seshadri K, Sadacharan D, Velayutham K, 2016, Fasting practices in Taamil Nadu and their importance for patients with diabetes, Indian J Endocrinol Metab, Nov-Dec, 20, 6, 858-862.

220    Taken from Trepanowski J, Bloomer R, 2010, The impact of religious fasting on human health, Nutrition Journal, 9, 57.

221    Trepanowski J, Bloomer R, 2010, The impact of religious fasting on human health, Nutrition Journal, 9, 57.

222    Taken from Trepanowski J, Bloomer R, 2010, The impact of religious fasting on human health, Nutrition Journal, 9, 57.

223    Nita M. 2019, 'Spirituality' in Health Studies: Competing Spiritualities and the Elevated Status of Mindfulness. J Relig Health. Oct;58(5):1605-1618.

224    Seamus Heaney, 2010, The Human Chain, London: Faber, 3.

225    deGraaff E, Bennett C, Dart J, 2024, Empathy in Nutrition and Dietetics: A Scoping Review, Journal of the Academy of Nutrition and Dietetics, Sep;124(9):1181-1205.

226    Ibid.

227    Rogers, CR, 1975, Empathic: An unappreciated way of being, J Counseling Psychol, 5, 2-10.

228    Kottler, J. A. (2010). On being a therapist (5th ed.). San Francisco, CA: Jossey-Bass.

229   Honig C, 2019, Thesis Compassion Fatigue in Registered Dietitians who treat patients with eating Disorders, Walden University ScholarWorks, https://scholarworks.waldenu.edu/cgi/viewcontent.cgi?article=9202&context=dissertations

230   deGraaff E, Bennett C, Dart J, 2024, Empathy in Nutrition and Dietetics: A Scoping Review, Journal of the Academy of Nutrition and Dietetics, Sep;124(9):1181-1205

231   Braddock J, 2019, Mental Health and the Registered Dietitian Nutritionist, Journal of Academy of Nutrition and Dietetics, 119, 12, 2109-2112

232   https://www.careerexplorer.com/careers/registered-dietitian/satisfaction/#:~:text=At%20CareerExplorer%2C%20we%20conduct%20an,the%20bottom%2026%25%20of%20careers.

233   Honig, 2019, Compassion Fatigue in Registered Dietitians who Treat Eating Disorder Patients, Walden College, https://scholarworks.waldenu.edu/cgi/viewcontent.cgi?article=9202&context=dissertations

234   Ross LJ, Mitchell L, Williams E, Lynch P, Munro J, Williams L, 2011, Impact of a resilience and wellbeing program: A longitudinal cohort study of student dietitians, Nursing and Health Sciences, 24, 591-600).

235   Langevin H, Berger A, Edwards E, 2023, Interface of resilience with other related concepts in physiological and psychosocial/spiritual domains, Stress and Health 39, S1, 10-13

236   Paal P, Helo U, Frick E, 2015, Spiritual Care Training Provided to healthcare professionals: A Systematic Review, Journal of Pastoral Care and counseling 69, 1, 19-30

237   Grzegoz J, Matzka D, 2024, The relationship between strength of religiousness, faith &in relation to post traumatic growth among nurses caring for Covid 19 patients in Eastern Poland, Front Psychiatry, Jan, 8, 14, 1331033

238   Muneeba A, 2019, Effect of spiritual intelligence on effective change management: a review of selected researches, Electronic Research Journal of Social Sciences and Humanities, 1,1, Jan-Mar

239   Oler JS, Nyland NK, 2005, The effect of religiosity and spirituality on work practice and trust levels in managers and their subordinates in food and nutrition care departments, Journal of American Dietetic Association, August 105, Supplement 8, 38

240   Hancock REE, Bonner G, Hollingdale R, Madden AM, 2012, "If you listen to me properly, I feel good': a qualitative examination of patient experiences of dietetic consultations, Journal of Human Nutrition and Dietetics, 25, 275-284.

241   Narayanasamy A, 1999, NET ASSET: a model for actioning spirituality and spiritual care education and training in nursing, Nurse Education Today, May, 19, 4, 274-85.

242   McSherry W, Ross L, 2002, Dilemmas of spiritual assessment: considerations for nursing practice, Journal of Advanced Nursing, July38, 5,479.

243   McSherry W, Ross L, Attard J, van Leeuwen R, Giske T, Kleiven T, Boughey A, Network E, 2020, Preparing undergraduate nurses and midwives for spiritual care: Some developments in European education over the last decade, Journal for the Study of Spirituality, 2002,10, 1, 55-71.

244   Baldacchino, D, (2015) Spiritual Care Education of Health Care Professionals, Conference Report, Journal of Religions, 6, 594-613.

245   Rykkje L, Bakstad Sovik M, Ross L, McSheery W, Cone P, Giske T, 2021, Educational interventions and strategies for spiritual care in nursing and healthcare students and staff: A scoping review, J Clin Nurs, 31, 1440-1464.

246   The Nursing and Midwifery Council, the Nursing and Midwifery Council in the UK Requirements for pre-registration nursing programme, London: NMC,

247   Strategy Lab for Higher Education, 2015, Indianapolis, IN, StrategyLabs. LuminaFoundation.org, from presentation given by Joellen Shendy, Registrar at University of Maryland University College, on November 18, 2015.

248   Fowler J, Streib H, Keller B, 2004, Manual for faith development research, available online, https://www.researchgate.net/publication/29871965_Manual_for_faith_development_research ,2019

249    Pucharlski CM, Larson D, 1998, Developing curricula in spirituality and
       medicine, Aca Med, 73, 970-974.

250    Mitchell C, Epstein-Peterson Z, Bandini J, Amobi A, Cahill J, Enzinger A,
       Noveroske S, Peteet J, Balboni T, Balboni M, 2016, Developing a Medical
       School Curriculum for psychological, moral, and spiritual wellness: student
       and faculty perspectives, J of Pain and Symptom Management, 52, 5, Nov,
       727-735

251    Balboni M, Bandini J, Mitchell C, Epstein-Peterson Z, Amobi A, Cahill J,
       Enzinger A, Noveroske S, Peteet J, Balboni T, 2015, J of Pain and Symptom
       Management, 50, 4, October, 507-515

252    Mallery S, Mallery P, 2022, Centers of value and the quest for meaning in
       faith development: A measurement approach, Frontiers in Psychology,
       Hypothesis and Theory, Sept ,28

253    Mitchell C, Epstein-Peterson Z, Bandini J, Amobi A, Cahill J, Enzinger A,
       Noveroske S, Peteet J, Balboni T, Balboni M, 2016, Developing a Medical
       School Curriculum for psychological, moral, and spiritual wellness: student
       and faculty perspectives, J of Pain and Symptom Management, 52, 5, Nov,
       727-735.

254    Viftrup DT, Nissen R, Søndergaard J, Hvidt NC. 2021, Four aspects of
       spiritual care: a phenomenological action research study on practicing and
       improving spiritual care at two Danish hospices. Palliat Care Soc Pract. Oct
       22;15

255    Balboni M, Bandini J, Mitchell C, Epstein-Peterson Z, Amobi A, Cahill J,
       Enzinger A, Noveroske S, Peteet J, Balboni T, 2015, J of Pain and Symptom
       Management, 50, 4, October, 507-515

256    Rykkje, 2021, Mitchell, 2016.

257    Bandin J, Thiel M, Meyer E, Paasche-Orlow S, Zhang Q, Cadge W, 2018, GSA,
       Annual Scientific Meeting 2, S1 cited in Rykkje L et al., 2021.

258    Hvidt, N. C., Nielsen, K. T., Kørup, A. K., Prinds, C., Hansen, D. G., Viftrup,
       D. T., Assing Hvidt, E., Hammer, E. R., Falkø, E., Locher, F., Boelsbjerg,
       H. B., Wallin, J. A., Thomsen, K. F., Schrøder, K., Moestrup, L., Nissen,

R. D., Stewart-Ferrer, S., Stripp, T. K., Steenfeldt, V. Ø., ... Wæhrens, E. E. (2020). What is spiritual care? Professional perspectives on the concept of spiritual care identified through group concept mapping. British Medical Journal Open, 10(12)

259 Viftrup DT, Nissen R, Søndergaard J, Hvidt NC. 2021, Four aspects of spiritual care: a phenomenological action research study on practicing and improving spiritual care at two Danish hospices. Palliat Care Soc Pract. Oct 22;15

260 Markham I, 1998, Spirituality and the world faiths. In the Spiritual Challenge of Health Care, Cobb M & Robshaw V eds, Churchill Livingstone, Edinburgh, 73-88

261 Armstrong K, 2019, The lost art of scripture-rescuing the sacred texts, Newsweek, Nov 11.

262 Pucharlski & Guenther, 2012.

263 McSherry W, Ross L, 2002.

264 Rykkje L, Bakstad Sovik M, Ross L, McSheery W, Cone P, Giske T, 2021, Educational interventions and strategies for spiritual care in nursing and healthcare students and staff: A scoping review, J Clin Nurs, 31, 1440-1464

265 USCCB, Coworkers in the Vineyard, 2005, Washington DC.

266 Rykkje, 2021.

267 Rhodes R, Smith L, "Molding Professional Character," Kenny N Shelson eds, Lost virtue: Professional Character Development in Medical Education (Elsevier, 2006).

268 Pucharlski & Guenther, 2012.

269 Cohen JJ, 2005, The work ahead: AAMC president address, November 6 2005 cited in Puchalski 2012.

270 Popovich Robert, Personal conversation with author, Oct. 10, 2024.

271 Wald, 2015.

272 Wald, 2015.

273 Puchalski, 2012.

274 Hilsman G, How to get the most out of clinical pastoral education (Jessica Kingsley Publishers, 2018).

275 Hilsman, 2018.

276 Meier DF, Morrison RS, 2001, "The inner life of physicians and care of the seriously ill," JAMA, 286: 3007-3014 in Mitchell 2016.

277 Hilsman 2018.

278 Ibid.

279 Ibid.

280 Ibid.

281 Mitchell, C Epstein-Peterson Z, et al., 2016, Developing a Medical School Curriculum for Psychological Moral, and spiritual wellness: student and faculty perspectives, journal of Pain and Symptom Management, 52, 4, 727-736.

282 Vifrup, 2021.

283 Hilsman, 2018.

284 Ibid.

285 Hilsman, 2017.

286 Popovich, 2024.

287 Wolfelt, 2007.

288 Hillsman, 2017.

289 Hilsman, 2017.

290 Hilsman, 2018.

291 Ibid.

292 Ibid.

293 Ibid.

294 Hilsman, 2018.

295 Balboni, 2016.

296 Hemenway, p. 215.

297  Hilsman, 2018.

298  Popovich 2024, personal conversation.

299  Sladdin I, Ball L, Gillespie B, Chaboyer W, A comparison of patients' and dietitians' perceptions of patient-centred care: A cross-sectional survey, *Health Expectations*, 2019, 22: 457-464.

300  Hilsman, 2018.

301  Ibid.

302  Hilsman, 2017.

303  Ibid.

304  Sulmacy, D, p 40.

305  Hilsman 2017.

306  Ibid.

307  Popovich, 2024.

308  Baldacchino, 2015.

309  Carlson L, Tamagawa R, Stephen J, Doll R, Faris P, Dirse D, Speca M, 2014, Tailoring Mind-Body Therapies to Individual Needs: Patients' Program Preference and Psychological Traits as Moderators of the Effects of Mindfulness-based Cancer Recovery and Supportive-Expressive Therapy in distressed Breast Cancer survivors, J Natl Cancer Inst Monogr, 50, 308-314.

310  From Association of Professional Chaplains, 6/1/2009, https://www.apchaplains.org/wp-content/uploads/2022/06/complementary_spiritual_practices.pdf

311  See Shelley Wood, "Regular Fasting May Improve CVD Risk," Medscape Medical News, Nove. 14, 2007 and Today's Dietitian, Vol 11, No 8, August 2009 issue.

Book Cover by Daniel Prescott-Bennett

Editing by Sophie Elletson

Edition 1 2025

www.ingramcontent.com/pod-product-compliance
Lightning Source LLC
Chambersburg PA
CBHW060803120626
46557CB00001B/66